KU-444-243

breastfeeding

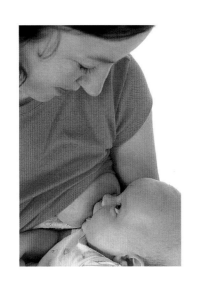

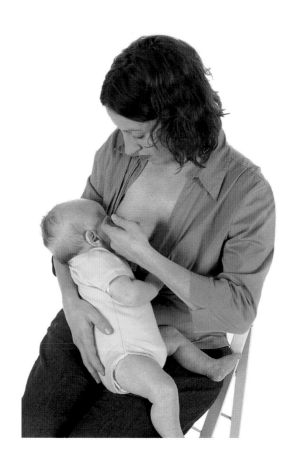

breastfeeding

nursing your baby and
introducing bottles

Jane Chumbley

hamlyn

contents

First published in Great Britain in
2003 by Hamlyn, a division of
Octopus Publishing Group Ltd
2–4 Heron Quays,
London E14 4JP

Copyright © Octopus Publishing
Group Ltd 2003

All rights reserved. No part of this
work may be reproduced or utilized in
any form or by any means, electronic
or mechanical, including photo-
copying, recording or by any
information storage and retrieval
system, without the prior written
permission of the publisher.

ISBN 0 600 60662 7

A CIP catalogue record for this book
is available from the British Library

Printed and bound in China

10 9 8 7 6 5 4 3 2 1

Safety Note: While the advice and
information in this book is believed
to be accurate, neither the author
nor publisher can accept any legal
responsibility for any injury or illness
sustained while following the advice
within it.

Introduction

If you have decided to breastfeed that is great news. By doing this you are giving your baby a real head start in life. Breastfeeding can be very rewarding, but it can take time to get used to it and you may have some hiccups on the way. That is where this book comes in. It is full of practical information, explanations, ideas and tips, plus helpful comments from women who have grappled with problems and found solutions. You can read it from cover to cover or section by section as you prefer. At the back there is a comprehensive index, a troubleshooting chart and some common questions and answers that will direct you to the help you need.

If you have not yet decided whether to breastfeed, then this book can help you take an honest look at what is involved. You may find chapter 1 particularly useful. If you have been breastfeeding and you want to start mixing in some bottles then you will find the help you need in chapter 6. Be reassured that 97 out of 100 women can successfully feed their babies – if they get help at the right time.

Good luck with your breastfeeding!

Problem-free breastfeeding: a checklist

Use this checklist to make sure you are doing all you can to help breastfeeding go well.

- Make it clear during labour – and on your birth plan – that you want to breastfeed.
- Feed your baby as soon as possible after birth.
- Feed on demand, day and night.
- Learn how to attach your baby to the breast (see pages 14–15).
- Get a specialist to check your feeding technique, even if you are not having problems.
- Avoid giving your baby formula milk in hospital.
- Do not give any bottles in the first 4 weeks.
- Make friends with your local breastfeeding counsellor.
- Get the support of your partner, parents and close friends.
- Be patient.
- Get help as soon as you suspect there may be a problem – do not wait until you know things have gone wrong.

Right: Breastfeeding your baby gives you plenty of opportunities to bond.

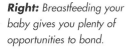

getting together

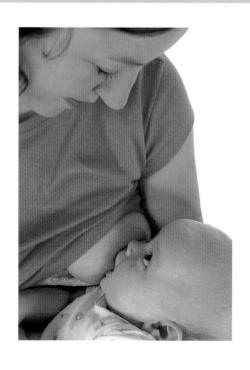

1

- Breasts and breast milk

- Getting into a good position

- Coming off and on the breast

- Breast refusal

- Problems in the early days

- Feeding bras

Breasts and breast milk

Breastfeeding can be physically demanding in the first few weeks: it takes time to get it right and you may feel that you have no sooner sorted yourself out after one feed than your baby is ready for the next. However, invest time now and you will save it in the future – making up bottles is not nearly as quick and convenient as breastfeeding, especially in the middle of the night or halfway through your weekly shop. Think of it as a skill you need to learn.

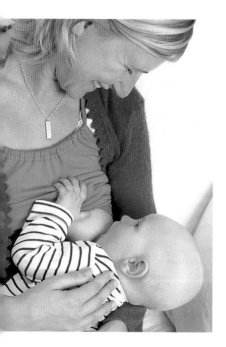

Above: Breast milk is the perfect food for newborn babies and a woman's breasts are designed to provide this milk.

Experts agree that breast milk is the best food for newborn babies. In fact, it is a perfect food – completely clean, packed with precious antibodies and containing just the right nutrients. What is more breastfeeding is good for women, protecting them against some serious diseases.

- Breast milk protects babies against diarrhoea, ear infections, urinary infections, eczema, diabetes, chest infections and obesity.
- Breast milk provides babies with substances that fight infection and support their developing immune system.
- Babies who are given nothing but breast milk for more than 3 months have been found to have a higher IQ than those given formula milk.
- Breastfeeding protects women against ovarian cancer, breast cancer and hip fractures.
- Breastfeeding uses up the fat stored during pregnancy.

Knowing how milk is produced can help you understand some of the initial problems you may be faced with.

Breast structure

A woman's breasts are designed to produce milk. Inside each breast there are about 20 lobes, each with its own duct system. The main duct branches out into smaller ducts that end in clusters of milk-producing cells called alveoli. The ducts widen into tiny reservoirs that hold a small store of milk, then converge on the nipple. Muscle cells surround the alveoli.

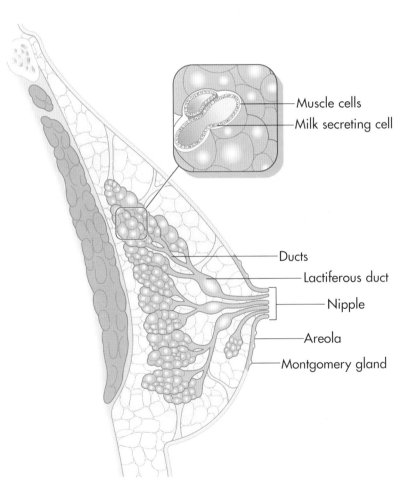

Muscle cells
Milk secreting cell

Ducts
Lactiferous duct
Nipple
Areola
Montgomery gland

Below

❶ The baby's stimulation of the nerve endings in the nipple sends more messages to the brain.

❷ The posterior lobe of the pituitary gland receives these messages and releases oxytocin which causes the muscle cells surrounding the milk-producing cells and ducts to contract.

❸ The contraction of the muscle cells propels the milk down the ducts to the nipple and into the baby's mouth. This is called the let-down reflex.

How breasts make milk: supply and demand

- The baby sucks at the breast and stimulates nerve endings. The nerves send messages to the brain telling it to release two hormones: prolactin and oxytocin.
- The prolactin stimulates the alveoli to make more milk. The oxytocin tells the muscle cells around the alveoli to contract, squeezing the milk into the reservoirs where the baby can get to it. (This squeezing is called the 'let-down' reflex.)
- The more the baby sucks, the more milk is produced: a simple case of supply and demand.

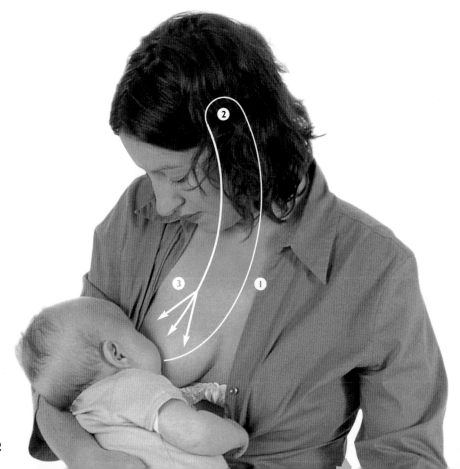

Facts about breastfeeding

- Size is irrelevant – you can breastfeed no matter how small your breasts.
- Ninety-seven per cent of women can breastfeed – even if your nipples are flat or inverted you can do it (see page 66).
- Lots of women who have had breast surgery will be able to breastfeed, although some may not (see page 67).
- You do not need to prepare your breasts for breastfeeding – they do that themselves.
- For the first day or two your breasts produce tiny amounts of a creamy-yellow substance called colostrum. This is all your baby needs until your milk comes in.

Types of breast milk

1 **Colostrum** is produced in the first few days. It is very rich in proteins and antibodies and very concentrated. In fact, the first feed may be only a teaspoonful. Colostrum lines your baby's gut and protects him against harmful bacteria. It gradually decreases when your milk comes in on days 3–5.

2 **Foremilk** is stored in the reservoirs and comes at the beginning of a feed. There is a lot of it and it is very thirst-quenching for your baby.

3 **Hindmilk** follows the foremilk towards the end of a feed. It is rich, creamy and full of fat-soluble vitamins – like a main course after a thin-soup starter. Babies need both foremilk and hindmilk.

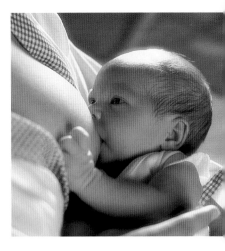

Above: The more your baby sucks at the breast the more milk is produced.

Getting into a good position

Over and over again you will read that breastfeeding problems start because the baby is not attached properly to the breast. If you can get this right from the beginning, you can avoid all sorts of difficulties.

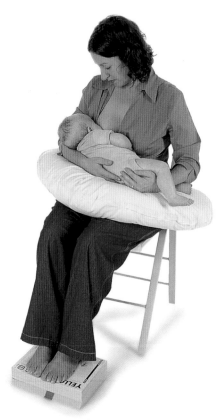

Above: Choose a comfortable chair which gives you firm support. You may find a low chair without arms is useful.

1 Sit upright with your back straight, your lap flat and your feet on a flat surface.

2 You may want to use a pillow or lapsack to take your baby's weight and to raise her just below the level of your breast.

3 Hold your baby with your right arm if you are feeding from the left breast (and vice versa). Her head, neck and back should be in a straight line, with the head tilted back slightly.

4 Support the base of her neck and head so that her neck is free to tip backwards as she moves her chin upwards.

5 Bring her body towards you and position her so that her nose is roughly in line with your nipple.

6 Gently touch your baby's mouth against your breast. Wait for her to open her mouth really wide, like a yawn.

7 When her mouth is open wide, move her to the breast quickly, with her chin leading and the nipple towards the top of her mouth. Her bottom lip should be aimed as far beneath the base of the nipple as possible, so that more of the underside of the areola (the brown-pigmented area around the nipple) is in her mouth. Her tongue should come forward over her bottom gums and her head should

not have to turn – you have a go at swallowing while you are looking over your shoulder!

8 When your baby is feeding well, you may change the supporting arm if you wish.

Latching on: a checklist
- Is your baby's mouth open wide?
- Is her chin up and pressed into your breast?
- Is her body in a straight line?
- Is her mouth covering the nipple and the areola underneath as well?
- Is your breast deep in her mouth?
- Are her lips spread wide?
- Is her nose free from your breast?
- Does she start sucking immediately, switching to long, deep sucks?
- Do her jaws move and her ears wiggle slightly during swallowing?
- Do you have eye contact?

Below: *To latch on well, a baby's mouth should be open wide so she gets a good mouthful of breast.*

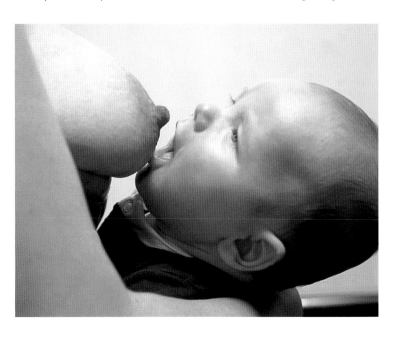

Tips on positioning

- If you are sitting in a deep chair, put plenty of cushions behind you to bring you forward.
- Put your feet on a low stool or a pile of telephone directories to make your lap flat.
- If your baby's arms flap around a lot, try wrapping them against her body.
- Move the baby to your breast, not your breast to the baby, otherwise you could get yourself into an awkward, uncomfortable position and your breast milk may not flow so freely.
- If your baby refuses to open her mouth wide, try gently brushing her top lip with your nipple or finger; this triggers a 'gape' reflex. It can take a few attempts to get this right to start with, so do not panic.
- Not all the areola needs to be in your baby's mouth. If you can see the areola, more should be

Below: *Once you have mastered feeding while sitting upright, try lying down.*

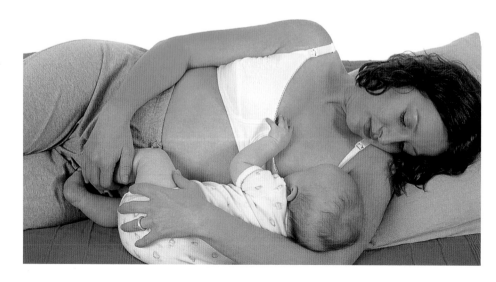

visible on top than underneath. You may need to get someone to check this for you because it is difficult to see the underside yourself.

- Do not squeeze or try to shape your breast. If necessary support it with your hand flat against your ribs.
- Feed on one breast for as long as your baby wants – after a break, offer the other.
- Once you have mastered feeding while sitting down, try lying down – this will make night-time feeds more comfortable.
- To release your baby from the nipple, put your little finger into the corner of her mouth to break the suction. Never pull your baby from the breast as it can hurt you!
- If you have any doubts about getting the correct position, see a breastfeeding counsellor before a problem develops.

'I found it very difficult to get any help at the hospital: the midwives were very busy and tended to just put Amy on the breast – they didn't have time to show me how to do it. When I got home it was a nightmare – I just couldn't get her in the right position. Fortunately there is a drop-in breastfeeding clinic where I live and the women there were brilliant – they told me what to do and then watched while I did it. I think I went every week for a month – just to check I'd got it right.'

Lisa Davies, mother of Amy (10 months).

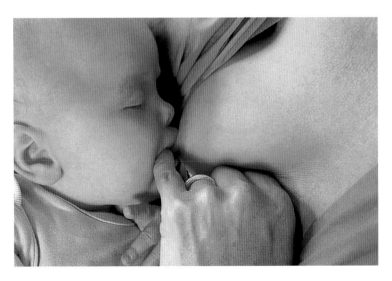

Left: Put your little finger in the corner of your baby's mouth to bring her gently off the breast.

Coming off and on the breast

Some babies find it difficult to get a good mouthful of the breast and tend to come off and on during a feed. This can be particularly difficult if your body has started to produce milk rather than colostrum: if your let-down reflex is in fine working order the milk can spray across the room! It can also be frustrating for your baby if he is enjoying his feed. If this happens regularly, there may not be enough suction to keep him latched on.

Counselling

If you are in hospital, you could ask to see a lactation consultant, although not all hospitals have these. However, a breastfeeding counsellor may visit the post-natal ward on certain days – ask the midwives to give you details. There are also organizations that you can ring for advice and there may be local breastfeeding counsellors or drop-in clinics that you can visit once you have left hospital.

- Get a breastfeeding counsellor to check your feeding position (see left).
- Concentrate on your baby during a feed and do not do anything else. The suction should be good enough for you to move without disturbing him but, for now, try to keep still.
- Check inside your baby's mouth for signs of thrush (see page 35). This can make his mouth so sore that feeding is uncomfortable.
- Check whether your baby is tongue-tied (see page 75).
- If your baby cannot seem to grasp the idea of feeding, he may need more time for his sucking action to mature, especially if he was born early. Also, in the early days, he may be feeling bruised and traumatized – especially if he was born by forceps or ventouse (suction cup).
- Express your colostrum or early milk into a lidless cup, and feed your baby from this (see page 19).
- Get specialist help.

Breast refusal

Some babies simply refuse to breastfeed. It's as if the sight of the breast really upsets them – this is called breast refusal.

The usual signs of breast refusal are arching of the back, screaming, and fighting with the hands as soon as your baby gets near the nipple. This may be due to any of several reasons:

- A slow let-down is making your baby frustrated.
- A forceful let-down is too much for your baby.
- Your baby is unable to breathe easily while he is feeding.
- Your baby has an unhappy memory of feeding – perhaps, in the early days, someone forced his head onto the breast and he was unable to breathe properly.

If the situation is desperate – if your baby hasn't fed at all for 6–8 hours, for example – you may need to express some milk, which can be given to him in a feeding cup. This will buy you some time to sort out the problem and prevent your breasts from getting over-full. If your baby has been feeding happily for some weeks and then suddenly refuses the breast, there could be other explanations (see page 40).

Let-down

Rates of let-down vary, and may sometimes lead to breast refusal.

- If your let-down is slow, express a little milk before you start to feed, to get it flowing.
- If your let-down is very strong, try lying back a little when you feed.

Cup-feeding

Newborn babies can lap milk, like a puppy, from a small feeding cup. This is ideal if you want to breastfeed but cannot for any reason – for example, if you are recovering from an operation or are finding it hard to establish breast-feeding and need a break. It means that your baby can receive your expressed breast milk in the early days without confusing the bottle teat with the nipple. All hospitals should have these cups, which are also available from retail outlets. Research has shown that using a cup takes no longer than using a bottle. Milk can also be given to your baby using a feeding syringe, spoon or a dropper.

Breathing

If you think breathing may be the problem:

- Check your feeding position. Is your baby's nose clear of the breast? If not, ask for help with positioning. You may be able to make your nipple more prominent by supporting your breast underneath – or your baby may need to be in a more upright position.
- Check that your baby's nose is clear. If it is clogged with mucus in the first day or so after the birth, the hospital staff should be able to clear it up for you. If it is blocked as the result of a cold, ask your doctor for some saline nasal drops, which will help to soften and clear the mucus.
- If your baby seems to cope with one breast but not the other, give her a feed on the easy side first, and then move her across without swinging her legs round – in other words, tuck her under your arm for the second breastfeed. If this seems to work, ask a lactation consultant or breast-feeding counsellor to watch you, so that she can suggest any changes for the long term (see also 'Refusing one breast', right).

Anxiety

If you think your own anxiety is the problem:

- Try to stay calm and do not panic.
- Have only one or two supportive people with you while you try to feed your baby. A crowd will make things worse.
- Wait until your baby is calm – do not try to feed her while she is screaming. You could try feeding her while she is still sleepy.
- Get her to suck on your little finger and then try to shift her onto the breast.
- Experiment with different feeding positions.
- Express a few drops of milk onto your nipple to tempt her.

Remember

Stay calm – your anxiety is easily off-set on to your baby.

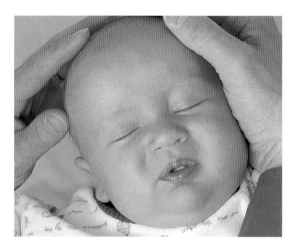

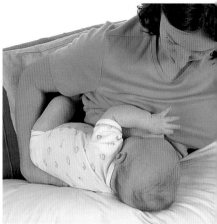

• Express some milk to be given in a cup so that you can both have a break.

Refusing one breast

If your baby refuses only one breast, it may be because your breasts or nipples are different, or that they have a different let-down reflex. Surgery or injury could have affected the nerves supplying the nipple or the number of milk ducts in a breast, for example.

Alternatively, she may have a pain on one side of her neck or in one ear. If necessary, you can feed on one side only, but you will find you become rather lopsided.

• Continue feeding from the breast that she accepts.
• Keep offering the other breast, using different positions, and express milk to keep up your supply on that side.
• Ask your doctor to check your baby over for signs of ear infection.
• Ask your doctor to give you a breast examination for any lumps.
• Consult a cranial osteopath (see page 58).

Above left: *Gentle massage from a cranial osteopath may help if your baby has a headache and feeding is difficult.*

Above right: *Experiment with different feeding positions if your baby seems to cope with one breast better than the other.*

Problems in the early days

Even if getting your baby latched on is fairly straightforward, you may have problems dealing with the increased size of your breasts and the sheer quantity of milk that they produce in the early days. You may also suffer from so-called 'afterpains', which make you tense up each time you start to feed. These are short-term problems but can be enough to put you off if you do not get the right kind of help and support.

Breast shells

Breast shells are ideal for collecting drips when you are feeding and if you sterilize the shell and a bottle you can collect the milk for use in a bottle or a cup-feeder. However, do not use a shell for more than 20 minutes and do not leave it in your bra between feeds – it will put pressure on your breast and could cause a blocked duct (see page 32).

Engorgement

About 2 or 3 days after your baby is born your breasts may get dramatically bigger, hot, hard and quite uncomfortable. This is called engorgement and is often referred to as 'your milk coming in'. It is caused by an increased blood supply to the breasts as full milk production gets underway. This is quite normal and no cause for alarm. It normally lasts only a few days but can be very painful. You may not be able to wear a bra or bear anything touching your breasts. Try the following remedies.

- Feed your baby as often as possible.
- If your breast is so full and hard that the nipple does not stand out, express a little milk before you start to feed: place a warm flannel on your breast, or take a warm shower or bath, and gently smooth the flat of your hand against your breasts to ease out some of the milk.
- Express a little milk using a hand pump.
- Put cold flannels on your breasts between feeds. The cold makes the blood vessels contract.
- Use warm or chilled thermal breast packs.
- Place chilled Savoy cabbage leaves inside your bra. They are thought to contain an enzyme that helps reduce swelling.

- Get help if you cannot get your baby to latch on to the breast properly; otherwise you could end up with sore nipples or a blocked duct (see pages 28–29 and 32).
- If your feeding bras do not fit, wear a soft night-time bra.
- Ask your doctor to prescribe you an anti-inflammatory drug.

Coping with leaks and squirts

Sometimes the let-down reflex is so powerful that your breasts work like a power shower (see right). Do not despair – you'll find this will calm down. In the meantime:

- Use the best-quality, most absorbent breast pads that you can afford and change them regularly.
- Always have a couple of muslin squares or terry nappies with you when you start to feed, to mop up spills.
- Try pressing the heel of your hand onto the nipple of the breast that you are not using; this can inhibit let-down.
- Put a breast shell inside your bra on the side you are not feeding from (see box, left).
- Do not put pressure on yourself by feeding in front of people before you and your baby have got used to it.

'To start with I found the let-down reflex really painful and very strong. If Katie came off the nipple the milk would squirt everywhere – three or four jets at a time. Sometimes it was funny but other times I got really fed up – it was really messy and put me off feeding in public for a long time. I also found the let-down worked in both breasts at the same time so I used to get very wet on the non-feeding side. Breast shells were a real life-saver.'

Wendy Thomas, mother of Katie (5 months).

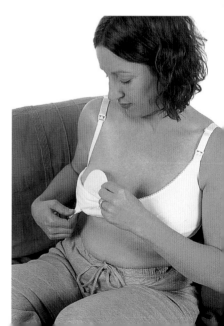

Right: *Use the most absorbent breast pads you can afford to cope with leaking between feeds.*

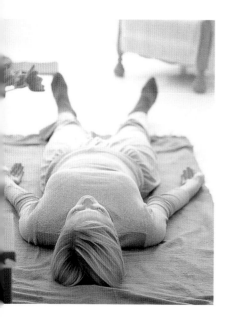

Above: *To help deal with afterpains, try to relax. Using techniques learned for labour might help.*

Frequent feeding

It is quite normal for babies to want to feed often after the first couple of days but, if feeds are less than 1 hour apart and happening 10 or more times a day after a week or so, there may be an attachment problem. If your baby suddenly starts feeding more frequently after a couple of weeks, he is probably having a growth spurt; this often happens after 2–3, 6 and 12 weeks. If he continues to be unsettled, he may be unwell.

- Ask a breastfeeding counsellor or lactation consultant to check your feeding position.
- During growth spurts, feed on demand to increase your supply.
- Check your baby for other symptoms, such as high temperature, and consult your doctor if you are unsure.

Afterpains

The hormone that causes the let-down reflex – oxytocin – makes the womb contract in labour, and the oxytocin released when you start to breastfeed can cause contractions again. These 'afterpains' vary from a dull ache to a full-blown contraction and can come and go for 5 or 10 minutes. Not all women get them, but they are quite normal and you should find that they stop after 4 days. They are usually more common, and worse, after second and subsequent babies.

Dealing with afterpains

- Use the relaxation techniques and calm breathing that helped you during labour.
- If you can anticipate a feed, take paracetamol 20 minutes beforehand, but do not take more than the maximum recommended dose.
- It is important to tell your midwife. Very occasionally afterpains happen because the womb is trying to push out a clot.

Feeding bras

There are several styles of feeding bra – you can find drop cup, zipped or front opening, for example. Drop-cup and zipped bras can be opened and closed with one hand, which can be an advantage, although you should be careful not to trap your skin in the zip.

Front-opening bras expose more of your breasts, which may be helpful when you are still learning how to get your baby well attached. Drop-cup bras may get damp if you have any leaks while you are feeding. You should not buy your feeding bras until you are at least 36 weeks pregnant. Some lingerie departments and bra agencies offer a fitting service. You will need a minimum of three bras, but do not wear them until you have had your baby – you can then exchange them if they are the wrong size.

Getting help

Although breasts are designed for feeding and babies need food, breastfeeding is not always as straightforward as we feel it ought to be. Just because your baby does not latch straight onto your breast and start sucking perfectly does not mean you are a failure – most women could do with some help. Do not be afraid to ask for help or to go on asking until you get the right help – the advice and support that makes it possible for you to feed your baby successfully.

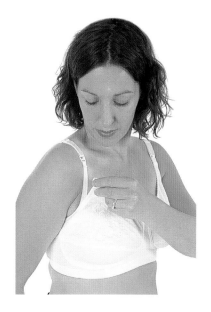

Above: *Drop cup feeding bras can be opened and closed with one hand to make manoeuvring your baby onto your breast much easier.*

ouch –
that hurts!

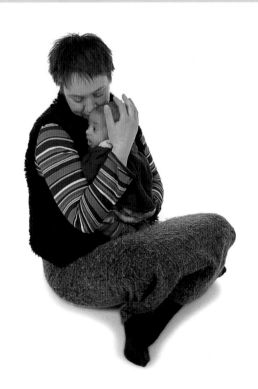

2

- Sore nipples

- Cracked and bleeding nipples

- Blocked ducts

- Breast abscess

- Thrush

Sore nipples

Breastfeeding should not be painful. When your baby is about 24 hours old your nipples may become very sensitive as the nerve endings are primed to respond to your baby's sucking. You may also find the let-down reflex uncomfortable at first (see page 12). However, once your baby is on the breast and feeding, it should be comfortable. Some women feel a pulling sensation in the breast, but again, it should not hurt.

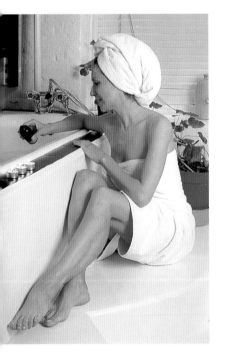

Above: *If you have very sore nipples you may be sensitive to soaps. Just use water to wash your breasts.*

If breastfeeding hurts then there is something wrong and you need to get help. Most problems with breastfeeding start because the baby is not properly attached to the breast. If possible, try to pre-empt these problems by seeing a breastfeeding counsellor or lactation consultant soon after your baby is born.

If your nipples are sore at the beginning of a feed in the first few days, there is probably nothing to worry about. This pain is probably the result of your breasts getting used to feeding and you will notice it less and less as the days go by. If the soreness goes on throughout the feed or if you notice that the nipple skin is red, bumpy, blistered, itchy or flaky, there is a problem. It could be:

- Your baby is not latching on to the breast properly, which may mean he is sucking for too long or putting pressure on the nipple.
- There is thrush in the baby's mouth.
- You or your baby are sensitive to creams or soaps.

It is important to do something straightaway in case the nipple cracks.

- Get an expert to check the way your baby is latching on to the breast.
- Try changing the feeding position – tucking the

baby under your arm rather than lying him across your lap, for example.

- Stop using any soaps, creams or sprays on your nipples. Just use water.
- At the end of a feed, express a little milk and let it dry onto the nipple – breast milk has healing properties.
- If you are using breast pads, change them after every feed.
- Check your baby's mouth for signs of thrush – white patches or spots that you cannot wipe away (see page 35). If this is the case, you will both need antibiotics.
- Never pull your baby off the breast. If you need to stop feeding, insert your little finger into the corner of his mouth to break the suction.

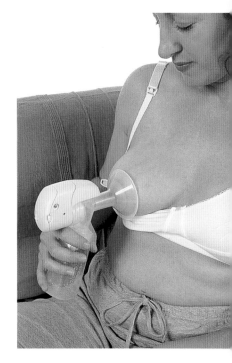

Above: *Expressing a little milk and letting it dry onto your nipple can help with healing.*

Cracked and bleeding nipples

If your nipple cracks, it may bleed every time you feed and scab-over between feeds. If you do not get help, you may find it painful each time you feed, so, if possible, speak to an expert before things get this bad.

'I was expecting breastfeeding to be really straightforward but I couldn't get Amy to latch on at all and by the end of day two my nipples were really sore and blistered. The pain was unbelievable and I spent most of the time in tears. It was only the breastfeeding counsellor who kept me going: we tried loads of things but what worked best was freezing a flannel and holding it on my nipples before I fed Amy. She also helped me get the feeding position right. It was agony, but it was worth it. After a week she was feeding really well.'

Fiona Harvey got off to a bad start when she was feeding baby Amy (now 2 years old).

If it has already happened then be assured that you can get through this: many women who are determined to breastfeed have continued and found a way to feed despite having cracked nipples. Cracked nipples usually happen because a baby is chewing on the nipple rather than sucking it into the back of her mouth. There are several things to try:

- Get an expert to check the way your baby is latching on.
- If possible buy some highly purified anhydrous lanolin ointment from the pharmacist and put it on your nipples after every feed until they have healed (see box, right). You could also use petroleum jelly to do this.
- Apply ice wrapped in a flannel to your nipples before feeding.
- Feed on the least sore side first (you may find you only need to give your baby a feed on one breast each time).
- People may suggest you try using nipple shields. These are made of thin latex and go over the nipple, and are designed so your baby can suck milk through them. However, they can make feeds take longer, and, because they restrict efficient emptying of the breast, can reduce your milk supply (hindering your baby's growth) or lead to illnesses such as thrush, breast abscesses or mastitis.
- Check your baby's mouth for signs of thrush. If she has thrush, you could get the infection in your

cracked nipple. If you suspect thrush, see your doctor for a prescription.
• If all else fails, express and rest for 24 hours. If a cracked nipple refuses to heal despite improving the way your baby latches on, the nipple may be infected. The treatment for this includes fusidic acid (an antibiotic) and paraffin gauze. If you have an infected nipple it will probably look wet, and may ooze pus.

Having a cracked nipple is very distressing. Talking to other women who have experienced the same problem and found a way through it can be encouraging – ask your breastfeeding counsellor if she can put you in touch with someone.

Moist wound healing

In the past women were advised to dry their cracked nipples after feeding but this means that a scab forms, which then comes loose during the next feed. This delays healing and extends the damage into the surrounding skin. It is better to keep the skin's natural moisture trapped inside so that healing can take place gradually. Using highly purified anhydrous lanolin will do this and also help relieve pain. Petroleum jelly is an alternative – apply a small amount after each feed. There is no hard research evidence to support the use of any creams for cracked nipples.

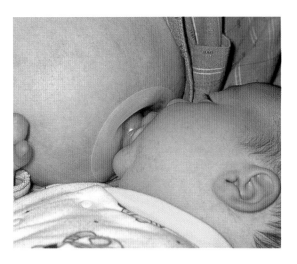

Left: Nipple shields can be used to protect sore nipples, but they carry risks and can reduce your milk supply.

Blocked ducts

If you develop a hot, red patch or sore lump on your breast and have hot, shivery, flu-like symptoms, you may well have a blocked duct. This means that a duct is not being emptied properly and milk is building up. This can happen when your milk first comes in if your baby is not attached properly. It can also be caused by pressure on one part of your breast – from a tight bra, a breast shell or a poor feeding position. A blocked duct may lead to non-infective mastitis (see right), so do not delay – you need to get the milk flowing.

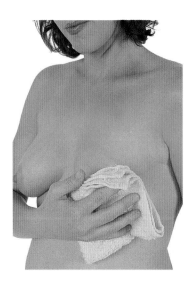

Above: *Holding a warm flannel over your breast before you feed may help with a blocked duct and relieve soreness.*

- Continue to feed your baby at every opportunity, starting with the lumpy breast – you will find that the problem will become worse if the breast gets over full.
- Check that your bra is not too tight – switch to a different bra if possible.
- Find a position in which your baby is actively feeding from the lumpy area. Try to point his chin towards the lump.
- Hold a warm wet flannel over your breast before you feed.
- Gently massage the lumpy breast while you are in the bath, stroking towards the nipple. You could use a wide-toothed comb dipped in baby oil. Massage helps to break up the lump.
- Gently massage your breast while feeding.

With early treatment, the blocked duct should get better within a few days. If it doesn't, you should consult a breastfeeding counsellor. If flu-like symptoms develop, you should see your doctor (see 'Mastitis', right).

Mastitis

There are two types of mastitis: infective and non-infective, both of which are inflammations. It feels like having a blocked duct, but you will also feel hot and shivery. Non-infective mastitis is caused by milk in a blocked duct leaking into your bloodstream, usually because your baby is not attaching properly. Your blood treats the milk as a foreign protein, producing the flu-like symptoms.

- Follow the advice for a blocked duct (left).
- Feed your baby as often as possible.
- Get as much rest as possible.
- Drink lots of water.
- Do arm-swinging exercises to boost circulation.
- Take paracetamol or ibuprofen.
- Consult your doctor if you are still feeling poorly after 12–24 hours.

Infective mastitis happens when bacteria get into the breast, often from your baby's nose or mouth. Testing for bacteria in a sample of breast milk is the only way to confirm it, but tends to take a long time. If increasing drainage from the breast does not help after 12–24 hours, the usual treatment is antibiotics, even though they can have side-effects (nausea, diarrhoea and thrush). Untreated mastitis can lead to a breast abscess (see page 34).

- Ask your doctor for an antibiotic that is safe for you to use, such as cephalexin or flucloxacillin.
- Eat live yoghurt while taking the antibiotic.

'The first time I had mastitis was the worst. My temperature went up and my breast was like a red, swollen balloon. I couldn't bear anyone to touch it and stopped feeding on that side. The midwife said I needed antibiotics, which I took, but the pain stayed and Tommy got diarrhoea. After a week I gave up breastfeeding altogether. I found out later that this was the worst thing I could have done.

'Next time it came I kept on feeding, and it worked. With my third baby I asked a breast-feeding counsellor for help, and she suggested I shouldn't wear a bra at night, or use breast shells in my bra during the day. I didn't have mastitis once with Henry.'

Jane Williams, mother of Tommy (6 years), Sally (4 years) and Henry (1 year).

Antibiotics: a warning

Antibiotics can be a very effective treatment for bacterial infection, but they can cause problems – some babies may get diarrhoea and nappy rash. They also wipe out the healthy bacteria that keep yeast infections such as thrush at bay.

Breast abscess

Although a breast abscess will make a lump in your breast it may or may not be painful. However, you are likely to feel ill, with symptoms like those of a blocked duct or mastitis. The difference is that you may see blood or pus in your breast milk or coming from your nipple.

Sore breasts

If your breasts are sore or breastfeeding is painful and there are no obvious problems, such as a cracked nipple or a lump, then you may have thrush in your milk ducts. This may feel like a deep, stabbing pain during and between feeds.

If this happens:
- See your doctor immediately. You will need antibiotics and the abscess may need to be lanced, drained or aspirated – where the pus is drawn off with a syringe.
- Ask your doctor about long-term antibiotic treatment as an alternative to aspiration (you will need to wait for a sample of pus or milk to be cultured to make sure you get the right antibiotic).
- Continue feeding. If your baby won't feed from the affected breast or if you find it too painful, just express milk from that side and feed on the other side.

If you have been receiving treatment for mastitis, and there is no improvement, it is worth asking your doctor whether you might have an abscess. Abscesses can form on the breast through unresolved long-term problems with attachment and milk drainage.

Thrush

Thrush is becoming quite common, and is easily passed between babies and mothers. It can cause many different problems so it is always worth considering if you are searching for a solution – although problems are more often the result of a poor feeding position. If you are prone to thrush and have had antibiotics or a cracked nipple, you need to be on the lookout for it every day.

Thrush action plan

1 Spot it. Look for white patches in your baby's mouth; nappy rash; red, sore, itchy, scaly nipples; nipple pain after pain-free feeding.

2 Attack it. Avoid soap; keep nipples dry; get acidophilus capsules from a pharmacy or health-food shop.

3 Get help. Your doctor or health visitor can prescribe miconazole antifungal cream for you and miconazole gel or nystatin drops for your baby. Both you and your baby should be treated at the same time.

4 Avoid it. Wash with water, not soap; eat live yoghurt; avoid antibiotics if possible.

5 Prevent the spread. Wash your hands and do not store expressed milk for use later – it could cause another bout.

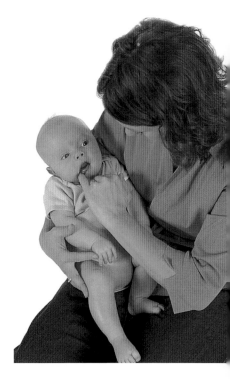

Above: You can check your baby's mouth for signs of thrush – look for white patches.

is my baby getting enough?

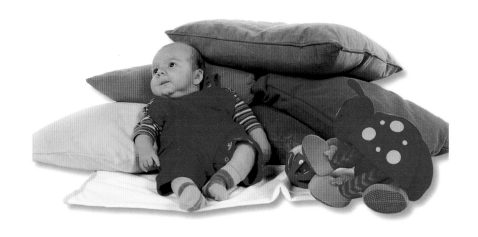

3

How much milk and how often?

When you are bottle-feeding everything is measured so it is easy to see exactly how much a baby has taken. With breastfeeding, it is not so simple. Some babies want feeding every 2 hours; others can go 4 hours between feeds.

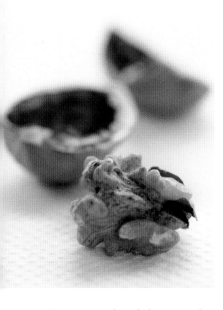

Above: *A newborn baby's stomach is the size of a large walnut – it doesn't take much milk to feel full!*

When you are breastfeeding you will find you have to use other ways of judging whether your baby is getting enough.
- Does he seem satisfied after a feed?
- Does he come off the breast of his own accord, and look 'stuffed'?
- Does he produce five or six wet nappies a day?
- Is he putting on weight?
- Is his skin soft and moist?
- Is the inside of his mouth moist and pink?

If the answer to all these questions is 'yes', your baby is getting enough milk. Otherwise, it is worth investigating further.

How much?

It is impossible to say precisely how much milk a baby needs: different babies have different needs and these change over time. To start with, your body produces colostrum – a rich, creamy-yellow substance packed with nutrients and antibodies. If you need to express colostrum for any reason – if your baby is in special care, for example – you might be surprised at how little there is: enough to fill a small syringe perhaps (see page 13). However, a newborn baby's stomach is only the size of a large walnut or a squash ball, so he does not need much to feel full.

When your milk has come in and breastfeeding is established, your breasts should produce as much milk as your baby needs. When your baby feeds it is as if he is ordering his next meal: the milk is made while he feeds and, if he is particularly hungry or his needs change, your breasts will respond by producing more as he sucks. After a month or two of breastfeeding, your breasts will learn not to make too much milk in advance and they will stop getting really full and heavy just before a feed.

How often?

Every new mother wants to know how often to feed her baby. This is not surprising since a new baby is a big responsibility and you want him to grow and be content. Unfortunately, there are no hard-and-fast rules. Long gone are the days when babies were fed every 4 hours – breastfeeding needs to be more flexible and it helps not to clock-watch. The following is a general guide.

- **Immediately after birth:** although babies are not hungry, this is a good time to start feeding.
- **Day 1:** babies are often sleepy in the first 24 hours and may only need to feed three times in this period.
- **Days 2–5:** as babies wake up they become more interested in feeding and may feed ten or more times over a 24-hour period. This helps to stimulate the milk supply and to relieve engorgement (see page 22).
- **End of first week:** babies may take possibly eight feeds in 24 hours.

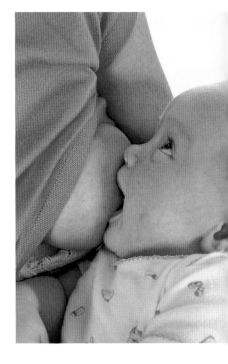

Above: As your baby becomes more awake and alert he will become more interested in feeding.

Reluctant feeders

What if your baby just does not seem interested in feeding? There are several reasons why this may happen in the early days.

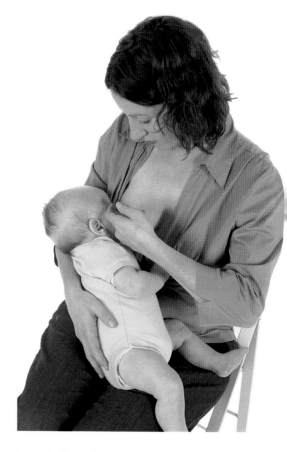

Right: If your baby is very sleepy you may need to keep her awake during a feed by stroking her cheeks or playing with her feet.

- **Sleepy baby:** a baby born more than 2 weeks early may not suck well and may tire easily.
- **Jaundice:** about one in two newborn babies has jaundice – as the immature liver struggles to process the products of normal red-cell breakdown there is a build-up of bilirubin in the blood, which produces yellowing of the skin and

the whites of the eyes. Babies do not need any treatment for this unless the bilirubin levels rise too high. However, jaundice can make a baby sleepy and reluctant to feed. You need to persevere and try to feed every couple of hours. As the liver matures the jaundice should resolve and, in the meantime, your baby needs the fluids she gets from your milk. Also make sure that you put your baby in the light – this will help to bring down the bilirubin levels. There is no need to give your baby water. (See also Jaundice in newborn babies, page 76).

- **Pethidine hangover:** if you took pethidine during your labour your baby could be sleepy and unresponsive for days as a result, particularly if it was given less than 5 hours before birth. Babies with a pethidine hangover are slower to root around and suck. Some research suggests that epidurals may leave babies unresponsive.
- **Uncomfortable baby:** see chapter 4.
- **Hypoglycaemia:** also known as low blood sugar, can be caused by too little feeding (see page 77). Of course, there may be no obvious reason at all. Clearly, the longer your baby goes without food, the more stressful this is for you and the more anxious you will become. Your baby will probably sense that anxiety and frustration, which will not help. You may also find that the hospital staff are reluctant to let you leave before your baby has had at least one good feed.

'When Simon was born the labour had been really long and I think we were both exhausted. The last thing I wanted to do was feed him. Simon seemed pretty happy to sleep and I was too. I had a side room in the hospital so I actually slept quite well the first day and I suppose it was about 6 or 8 hours after he was born that the midwives started asking if I'd fed him. I did try but he wasn't interested – he'd suck for a bit and then fall asleep again. It was like that for the first 24 hours really – then they started to get really insistent. They stood over me while I tried to get him on and I got really nervous. Then they tried to put him on and he screamed and it was awful – I ended up in tears. After another day battling with it I just gave up and gave him a bottle which he took straight-away. Later I felt really cheated – I'm sure there was a reason why he was sleepy and with time we would have got there. I just wasn't confident enough at the time.'

Julia Evans, mother of Simon (9 months).

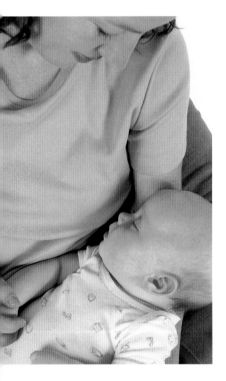

Above: *Try to get your baby wide awake before you start feeding by playing with him and talking to him.*

Encouraging a reluctant feeder

There are several things you can do to encourage your baby to feed.

- Get him wide awake before you start feeding: cool him down, play with him, talk to him.
- Try to keep him awake during a feed: talk to him, stroke his cheek, play with his hands and feet.
- If he does fall asleep and come off the nipple, sit him up, pat his back, wake him up and start all over again.
- Ask a breastfeeding expert to watch you as you get him latched on. She may spot something in the way the baby attaches to the breast that suggests why he finds feeding uncomfortable.
- Express colostrum by hand and use a feeding syringe, which the hospital will provide. This will give your baby food and stimulate your breasts.
- Ask if a paediatrician can check the baby again while you are in hospital. This is for reassurance that your baby is not ill.
- If you had pethidine during labour ask if your baby can have an injection of naloxone – an antidote that should stop him being over-sleepy in the first 48 hours. Also give your baby more time: do not hurry him, and do not let anyone force him onto the breast.

Frequent and lengthy feeders

Some babies like to suck and take an hour or more to finish a feed. Sometimes you may enjoy this and it is a good way of making sure you can sit down and relax! However, you may find it can be very draining, particularly if you want to do other things. So, why do some babies feed for such a long time?

It is possible that it is taking your baby a long time to get to the fat-rich hindmilk because he is not positioned properly on the breast (see chapter 1). Alternatively, he may just be enjoying the sucking sensation and the closeness he experiences when he is snuggled up with you.

To some extent it is up to you whether this is a problem or not. If it is, you could:
• See a breastfeeding expert to check your baby's attachment is correct.
• Put something in his cot, pram or basket that smells of you and your milk – a T-shirt or a handkerchief, for example.
• Try giving a dummy between feeds – but not for the first month or so, if possible (see note: page 62).
• Put him in a sling and carry him around between feeds. He will still be close to you and will be able to smell your milk.

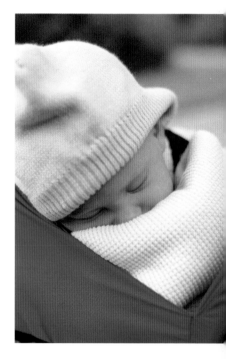

Above: If your baby wants to be close to you all the time, invest in a sling and carry him around between feeds.

Growth

In order to work out whether your baby is putting on enough weight, it is important to make the proper comparisons.

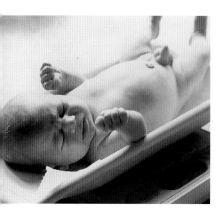

Above: *Your baby will be weighed regularly, but don't panic if she doesn't gain weight quickly.*

Slow growth

Babies quite commonly do not put on as much weight as quickly as the health professionals would like. Although this may prove not to be a problem, it leaves some women feeling anxious, guilty and powerless. Depending on the kind of advice and support you get, it can also undermine your confidence in breastfeeding, making you feel like giving up and resorting to formula milk – or at least topping-up with bottles of formula. Nevertheless, breast milk is highly nutritious and should give your baby all she needs, so why is this happening?

- Your baby may be nipple-feeding rather than milking the breast. If so, she will not be getting the fat-rich hindmilk, only the watery foremilk stored in the reservoirs.
- She may have been ill or slow to start feeding (see page 40).
- She may not be feeding frequently enough.
- She may have a medical condition.
- She may be settling into the weight-gain pattern that is right for her.

So what can you do if you feel concerned or under pressure from health professionals?

- Ask a breastfeeding expert to check your feeding position and the way your baby is attaching.
- Make sure your baby is always weighed naked and at roughly the same time after feeding – a 110g (4oz) feed can make a huge difference in a small baby's weight.
- Treat all gains since her lowest weight measured as weight gain – do not use birthweight as your marker for this.

Dehydration signs

A dehydrated baby can become very ill so it is important to look for the signs:

- Feed more frequently to increase your baby's intake and build up your supply.
- Express milk to stimulate your breasts into producing more.
- Take into account your baby's general health as well as weight gain. If she seems happy and her skin looks healthy, there may be no reason for you to be concerned.
- If your baby is vomiting after feeds there may be a specific problem, such as cow's milk intolerance (see page 60) or a condition called pyloric stenosis (see page 57).
- Give yourself time, and try not to panic.
- Ask if your health visitor could access growth charts based on breastfed babies. These show that, although totally breastfed babies may be heavier in the first few weeks, they are then overtaken by formula-fed babies; therefore it is not unusual for a breastfed baby to drop back a growth curve.
- Surround yourself with helpful people who support your decision to continue breastfeeding, for example by regularly attending a breastfeeding drop-in clinic.
- Ask your doctor if it is possible for your baby to be tested to rule out any medical conditions such as cystic fibrosis or coeliac disease (sensitivity to gluten).

Dehydration signs

A dehydrated baby can become very ill so it is important to look for the signs:

- **Lethargy • Weak cry**
- **Dry mouth • Dry eyes**
- **The soft spot on the head (the fontanelle) is sunken.**

If you think your baby is dehydrated see a doctor immediately.

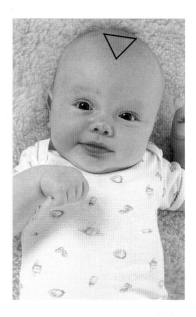

Above: If the fontanelle (soft spot on the head, indicated above) is sunken, this can be a sign of dehydration.

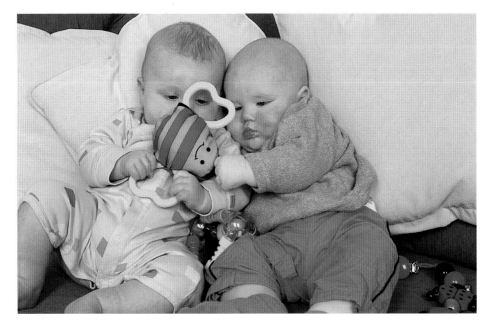

Above: *Babies double their birth-weight by 6 months and triple it by a year.*

Facts about growth

1 In the long term length or height is a better indicator of growth than taking a weight measurement, so it is worth making sure that you get accurate baseline measurements of your baby's length when he is both 10 days old and 6–9 months old.

2 In the first week or so it is quite normal for a baby to lose up to 10 per cent of his birthweight, although exclusively breastfed babies do not normally lose quite this much. He should regain any loss by the end of the second or third week.

3 Babies are expected to double their birthweight by 6 months and triple it by a year.

4 Babies should grow by around 25–30cm (9–12in) in the first year.

5 The growth charts in your baby's record book act as a guide. It does not matter which curve is being followed – all are within the normal range. The important thing is that, over time, your baby should be gaining weight and following one of the curves. Moving up or down one or two curves between measurements is not significant; it is the overall trend that counts.

6 Bottle-fed babies may put on slightly more weight than breastfed babies – an average of 140–200g (5–7oz) per week in the first 4 months compared to 110–230g (4–8oz) – but, as you can see, there is a wide range.

Left: Bottle-fed babies may put on more weight than breastfed babies.

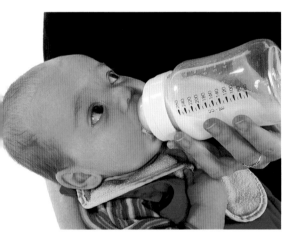

'My second son Matthew fed very well but he didn't regain his birthweight by day 14 and the midwives wouldn't sign him off. They kept coming with different scales and after 3½ weeks the health visitor was weighing him every 3 days because he'd only gained a few ounces. At 11 they said he was failing to thrive and that I must give him a bottle every 2 hours. But he didn't want to feed that often! In the end I complained to my doctor who declared Matthew perfectly healthy. I feel there was too much emphasis on charts and not enough on general health.'

Christine King, mother of Matthew, aged 7

47

Too little milk?

It is extremely unlikely that you cannot make enough milk for your baby. So what has put this idea into your head?

- **Is it because your breasts are small or feel soft?** After several weeks of feeding, your breasts will adjust and stop producing masses of milk in advance of a feed – they simply start making it as your baby feeds. As a result, they will feel empty. Similarly, if you have been feeding on and off all day or all evening, your breasts will not contain a huge store but they will still make milk as you feed. Most women feel less full in the evening than during the day. Small breasts are never a barrier to successful breastfeeding.
- **Is your baby failing to gain weight?** There could be many reasons for this (see page 44), and she may just be a small baby.
- **Do other babies seem bigger and other women's breasts seem leakier?** Do not make comparisons –

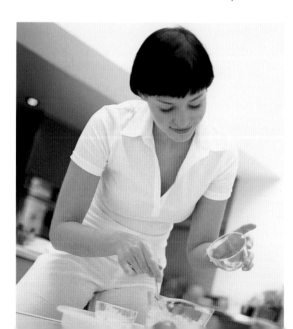

Right: Eating more during the day may help to improve your milk supply.

we are all different. If your breasts do not leak, just be thankful!

- **Has someone said something about it?** Do not believe all you are told. Ask an expert, such as a breastfeeding counsellor.
- **Does your baby never seem satisfied?** She may just be very hungry, comfort sucking or uncomfortable for some other reason (see page 50).
- **Is your baby very big?** Whatever your baby's size, you will produce enough milk to satisfy her needs until she is 6 months old. Of course, feeding a big baby can be demanding, so you may decide to wean her onto solids at 4 or 5 months, but do not feel under pressure to do this.
- **Do you find it hard to express milk?** This can be hard, and the amount you get is not related to your milk supply.

There are several reasons why your body might not make as much milk as it could:

- **Let-down failure:** in theory, being very anxious or tense as you feed might affect the let-down reflex that gets milk flowing. It may also fail if your baby is not properly latched on.
- **Supplementary feeds:** giving your baby extra water or bottles of formula will reduce your milk supply. Bottle teats require less jaw movement to produce milk and can weaken a baby's sucking, thus stopping her sucking strongly on the breast.
- **Illness:** being unwell might affect your milk in theory, but in practice mothers successfully breastfeed through famines and malnutrition.
- **Growth spurt:** if your baby is having a growth spurt, it may take a few days for your body to catch up with her increased needs.
- **Milk cells and ducts not developed properly:** this is very rare. Women with this so-called 'primary lactation failure' do not notice any breast changes during pregnancy and do not feel their milk coming in. They can still breastfeed, although their babies may need other milk as well.

How to improve your milk supply

- Get a breastfeeding expert to check the way your baby latches on.
- Cut out all other sources of milk or water.
- Increase the number of times you feed your baby and the length of feeds.
- Eat more yourself – a sandwich mid-morning, a banana mid-afternoon and a milky drink before bed.
- Feed fully on one side, then switch to the other and, if necessary, back again.
- Express a little milk and massage your breast with a warm flannel before a feed to get the let-down going.
- Cut out caffeine and alcohol if you suspect your let-down is not working.
- Express milk in the morning to be given as a top-up bottle after you have fed on both sides in the evening.

unhappy babies

- Why do babies cry?

- Wind

- Colic

- Vomiting

4

- Headaches and other pains

- Coping with crying

- Cow's milk intolerance

- Biting and fighting the breast

Why do babies cry?

If this is your first baby and you have had no close contact with any new babies before, you may not know what to expect in terms of crying behaviour. Is it normal for babies to cry for 2 or 3 hours in the evening? Should they sleep between feeds? Do they always scream until they are bright red in the face?

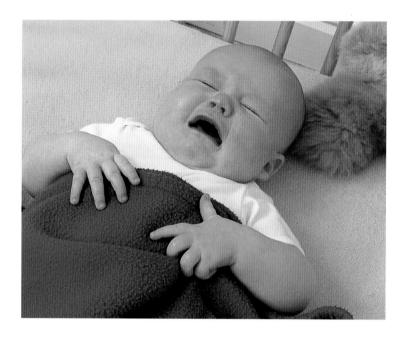

Above: *There are many reasons why babies cry – it may be time for some detective work!*

Babies are as individual as you and I, so you cannot expect your baby to behave in the same way as any other. However, this does not mean that you should put up with constant crying or niggling. It is quite common for breastfed babies to want more frequent feeding in the evening, because that is when the milk becomes more concentrated and satisfying. Some babies cry for 2 hours or more in the evening and others scream a lot, whereas a lot of babies sleep between feeds, especially in the early weeks, or are fairly settled and calm. If your baby is not one of the latter there may be something you can do about it. If you have any doubts about your baby's behaviour, talk to your health visitor, who knows the range of what is normal and what is not. Keeping a record of their crying episodes will help you to look at the situation objectively.

Dealing with an unhappy newborn baby is very demanding, both emotionally and physically. Constant crying and whingeing is upsetting, frustrating and disappointing. If you are breast-feeding and finding it a struggle, it is very easy to blame this for your baby's problems and your unhappiness. It is also true that, if you switch to bottles, other people can share the load and you can get more rest. On the other hand, breastfeeding may not be the root of the problem and, if it is, there may be a simple solution that does not involve giving up – a decision you may regret later on.

Crying is your baby's way of telling you that something is troubling her. Is she:
• Hungry?
• Too cold or too hot?
• Wet?
• Lonely or bored?
• Suffering from wind or colic?
• Suffering from headache or other pain?
Dealing with the first three problems is quite straight-forward, unless you are having problems getting your baby to latch on and take milk (see 'Getting into a good position', page 14). If so, then dealing with this problem is your number one priority – speak to someone today! If your baby's problem is wind, colic or a headache, then making changes to your breastfeeding may help (see pages 54–56 and 58). If your baby is bored, he may need some more stimulation.

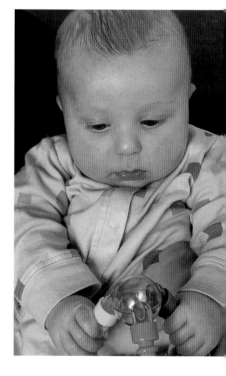

Above: Your baby may be bored, and need more stimulation.

Wind

Dealing with wind should be a fairly straightforward affair, although some babies seem to struggle with it and have more problems than others.

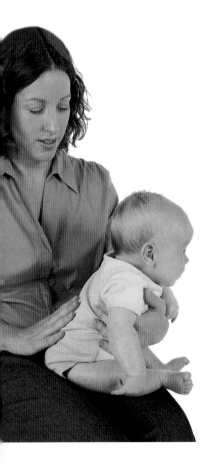

Above: Press or rub your baby's back with your hand to help dislodge wind.

When we say a baby has wind, what we really mean is that he has swallowed some air, which is now trapped like a little bubble in his tummy or digestive system, causing him pain.

The idea is to get him to bring up the wind and burp. You can do this by sitting him on your lap with the palm of one hand on his stomach, supporting his head between your outstretched thumb and first finger, and with your other fingers under his arm. It is the slight pressure of your hand on his tummy that should dislodge the wind, but you can press or rub his back with your hand.

Alternatively you can lay him over your shoulder and rub his back while his tummy is pressed against your shoulder or lay him down along the length of your arm or in your lap – you might want to save this until you feel more confident handling your baby. Whichever position you use, have a muslin square or terry nappy handy – burps tend to bring squirts of milk with them.

In hospital you may be told you should wind your baby after every feed. To be honest, this is not really necessary unless your baby has wind. See how you get on.

If you think your baby has a lot of wind:
• See a breastfeeding counsellor: if your baby does not have a good latch on the breast, he may be taking in air as he feeds. A change of position may do the trick.
• Avoid using bottles: bottle-fed babies tend to get more wind as they suck on the teat.

Colic

Having wind is not the same as having colic. Although trapped wind can be very painful it is unlikely to cause the very extreme discomfort colicky babies appear to experience. So, what is colic?

Actually, no-one is exactly sure what colic is. A common definition in medical circles is excessive crying in otherwise healthy thriving infants occurring for at least 3 hours a day, three times a week or more. In practice this means inconsolable crying that turns into a screaming fit, often during the late afternoon or early evening. Babies with colic typically draw up their knees, clench their fists and arch their backs in pain. They seem desperate to feed but may reject the breast after a few seconds and become even more distressed. Or they may feed, fall asleep briefly and then wake with more screaming. Colic does not normally start until the baby is about 1 or 2 weeks old but it can last for 3 months, sometimes more. It may disappear at 12 weeks or it may develop into a good-day/bad-day pattern until it stops. A number of babies still suffer from colic at 4, 5 or 6 months. It is estimated that one or two babies out of ten will have colic.

What causes colic?

Some doctors believe that colic is the result of the baby's intestines not working smoothly. Instead of contracting rhythmically to move food along, the intestines go into spasms that cause a lot of pain. It is unlikely that wind in itself is the cause of the problem, although there is no doubt that a screaming baby will swallow a lot of air, which can make the problem worse because the air gets trapped in the loops of the intestine during spasm. Babies may also feel better after a good belch. It is

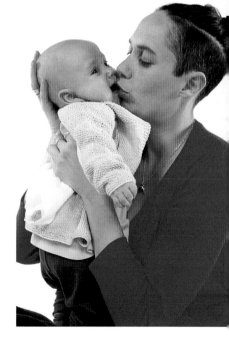

Above: *Colicky babies may scream for hours at a time and need a lot of love and attention.*

55

'My baby Josh always brought back some of his feed right from the start, but as time went on it got no better and we did worry. I stopped breastfeeding, thinking he would get on better with formula but that didn't work. In the end we took him for tests and the doctors discovered a problem with his stomach, which has to be maintained until he is old enough to have surgery.'

Belinda Gria, mother of Josh, aged 2 years.

Below: *Not all crying is caused by colic: try soothing your baby by stroking her cheeks and talking softly.*

also possible that some colic can be blamed on sensitivity to certain foods (see page 60).

Could breastfeeding be to blame? It may be hard to believe that there is a feeding problem if your baby is piling on the pounds and your nipples are not sore, but in some cases colic can be caused by poor positioning, leading to something called temporary lactose overload. This is more likely if your baby produces a lot of green, watery nappies and passes a lot of wind – top and bottom. Lactose is a sugar in breast milk that needs to be broken down by an enzyme called lactase. If it is not broken down, it passes into the lower bowel, where it is fermented by bacteria, producing gases and lactic acid (hence the wind and green nappies).

What may be the answer?

The solution may be to slow down the rate at which milk passes through the baby's gut, thus allowing time for the lactose to be broken down. The way to do this is to make sure your baby gets a good amount of the fat-rich hindmilk at each feed. If you have been offering both breasts at each feed, it is possible she is just getting foremilk – the watery milk that comes first. Increase the time that she has on the first breast to ensure that the hindmilk has come through.

A breastfeeding counsellor can also help by suggesting small alterations to the way your baby latches on and drains the breast when feeding. Research has shown that this can be very effective.

- Feed fully on one breast at each feed – particularly if you have a lot of milk. If your baby comes off the breast, sit her up and change her nappy if necessary, then offer the same breast again.
- See a breastfeeding counsellor, who can check your feeding position.

Vomiting

It is normal for babies to bring back – or posset – small amounts of milk after a feed. They may do this as soon as you bring them upright, when they burp or after they have been crying a lot. Occasionally even a perfectly healthy baby may vomit a more substantial amount – simply because they have taken in too much or have had a lot of wind.

However, regular or projectile vomiting is not normal and always needs to be investigated. It could be the result of:

- **Gulping too much air:** if your milk flow is very fast, express some foremilk before a feed.
- **Illness:** check for other symptoms, such as high temperature and diarrhoea, and see your doctor.
- **Gastro-oesophageal reflux:** in this, the stomach's contents flow back into the oesophagus. This is fairly unusual in breastfed babies and does not need any treatment as long as the baby is gaining weight and does not seem unhappy.
- **Cow's milk intolerance:** see page 60.
- **Pyloric stenosis:** about one in two hundred boys and one in a thousand girls has this fairly unmistakable condition. It causes projectile vomiting, with the vomit travelling up to a metre. It usually starts after about 2 or 3 weeks and is the result of a muscle overgrowth at the exit to the stomach. Until it is treated, the vomiting gets worse and the baby could be constipated and very dehydrated as well. An operation to correct the problem is very successful.
- **Other conditions:** hiatus hernia or strangulated hernia, where a small part of the bowel becomes trapped, will need an operation.

'I never really got to the bottom of it but I do know I produced huge amounts of milk with a very powerful let-down and Sally had very green nappies on the days when she was worst with her crying. Things improved a lot when she was having solids as well as milk – perhaps because my milk production calmed down or because she was feeding less often. It was a difficult few months but I would never regret my decision to breastfeed because she's been a very healthy toddler, with no ear infections or allergies and I'm sure that's because of the breast milk.'

Jane Fox's daughter had what she calls 'raging colic' at all times of the day for the first 4 or 5 months.

Headaches and other pains

Babies can't tell us when and where they are experiencing pain and it's only after successful treatment that parents are able to pinpoint the problem.

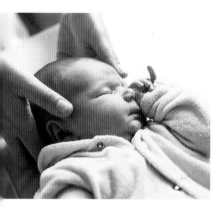

Above: A cranial osteopath gently manipulates the baby's skull to ease compression.

When a baby is born vaginally the plates of the skull overlap each other to make the baby's passage down the birth canal easier; this is called moulding. Some therapists – called cranial osteopaths – believe that this moulding may give the baby a headache.

If so, your baby may find it painful to lie down and you may always have trouble getting him to sleep in his basket or bed, although he may be quite happy lying on your chest. Moulding can also cause or aggravate colic or make feeding uncomfortable because the nerves supplying the stomach and the tongue both emerge from the skull behind the ear – an area that is often compressed during birth. If it remains compressed, this could interfere with feeding and digestion.

If you suspect this may be a problem:

- **See a cranial osteopath:** a cranial osteopath works by manipulating the baby's skull with extremely gentle movements to ease compression. If this is going to work there is often a dramatic improvement after the first or second visit, with further improvements after subsequent visits. An appointment lasts 30–60 minutes.
- **See a breastfeeding counsellor:** if your baby is uncomfortable feeding in a certain position, you may be able to help him by using a different position – putting his body under your arm, for example.

Coping with crying

If your baby cries a lot, you will need several strategies to get you through this difficult time.

There are a number of things you can do to help you cope with crying.

- **Earplugs:** these dull the sound and make it more bearable.
- **Go for walks:** the exercise will make you feel better and the jolting motion of the pram may soothe your baby.
- **Keep a diary** recording times and duration of crying, what you tried and how your baby reacted: over time you can see whether there is a pattern and you can tell when things are starting to improve.
- **Carry your baby in a sling:** this may not reduce crying but it means that you can stay close to your baby and rock him while being free to do other things.
- **Swaddle your baby:** some babies find it very comforting to be wrapped tightly in a blanket, perhaps because it reminds them of being enclosed in the womb.
- **Let your baby suck your finger or give him a dummy:** sucking is often very comforting for colicky babies (but see box: 'Dummies and breastfeeding', page 62).
- **Cut out coffee, tea and cola for 2 weeks:** see if it makes a difference.
- **Have a break:** get someone else to take charge while you go out.

Remember that crying can be a sign of an ear infection or other illness so see your doctor to get your baby checked over.

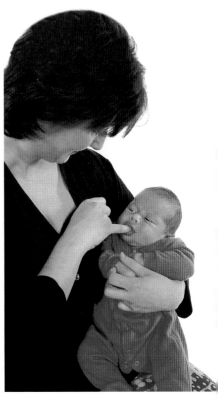

Above: Let your baby suck your finger if he has colic; it is often very comforting.

Cow's milk intolerance

There is some dispute about the extent of cow's milk intolerance in babies and young children. Many people believe it is diagnosed too frequently, and that babies' (and mothers') diets are restricted unnecessarily.

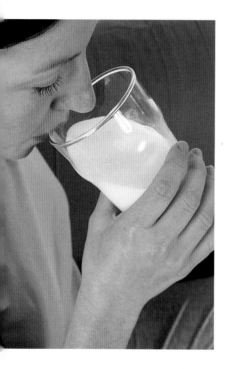

Above: Consult a dietician if you suspect your baby is intolerant to cow's milk in your diet.

It is very important to talk to a dietician before you jump to any conclusions or start modifying your diet in any way. It is true that some babies seem to have an allergic response to cow's milk that sends their guts into spasm – causing colic-type symptoms and vomiting. These babies may also fail to put on weight and suffer from eczema, asthma and allergic rhinitis (persistent runny nose). An intolerance to cow's milk is more likely if there is a history of atopic allergy (eczema, asthma, hay fever) in your family, or if your baby is given any formula milk, which is made with cow's milk protein, in the early days. A really sensitive, fully breastfed baby might react to cow's milk in his mother's diet.

What can you do?

- You can test for milk intolerance by fully breastfeeding and excluding all dairy products from your diet for at least 2 weeks. Talk this through with a dietician first (your doctor can refer you) to make sure you are left with a diet that meets your needs and those of your baby. A breastfeeding counsellor should be able to give you a cow's-milk-free diet sheet for breastfeeding mothers, which you may find helpful. You may want to avoid soya milk at the same time because it can induce allergic reactions in babies allergic to cow's milk and it is low in calcium. Goat's milk is an alternative (although this must not be given directly to babies).

- If your baby's symptoms improve or disappear while you are cutting out cow's milk, you will need to decide whether to continue breastfeeding and to cope with this diet in the medium term. Try drinking a glass of milk every 4 weeks to see if it produces any reaction. Usually this kind of intolerance is temporary.

- If you find that you cannot cope with the restricted diet and decide to switch to bottle-feeding, you will need to get a hypoallergenic formula, possibly on prescription from your doctor. This has been treated so that the proteins are partially digested, which means there is less stress on the baby's digestive system.

- An alternative might be to drink three bottles of an active yoghurt each day. Early results from a small study suggest that this may be enough to enhance the mother's immune system and stop the absorption and excretion of proteins into the breast milk. When it works, the result is apparently quite dramatic – usually within 24 hours of taking it.

Was it something I ate?

It is easy to blame yourself when your baby has a crotchety day. However, it is probably nothing to do with you. Everything you eat and drink gets into the breast milk, the amounts involved are very small. There are no foods that you must avoid or that have been consistently linked to colic or general fussiness in babies. Occasionally food or drink may cause a problem if it is unusual for you – garlic or highly spiced foods, for example – or you have it in excess – alcohol or caffeine, for example. More than five 140ml (5oz) cups of coffee a day could make a baby fussy. If there is a family history of allergies then your baby is more likely to react to certain foods. Soft cheeses are considered safe for breastfeeding because the Listeria bug is unlikely to pass into your baby's gut and the baby has your antibodies.

Biting and fighting the breast

Having your nipple bitten by a baby is no joke (she does not need teeth to hurt). So, do not encourage her by laughing, even in shock.

Dummies and breastfeeding

As far as breastfeeding is concerned, dummies have three possible drawbacks:

- They can mean a baby loses interest in sucking on the breast, which is not a good thing if your baby is a poor feeder.

- They may confuse a breastfed baby because they have a very different shape to the breast – even nipple-shaped dummies are not like a breast with its areola. Your baby's mouth makes a very different shape as it sucks on a dummy, so it may not be a good idea to use a dummy until breastfeeding is really well established.

- They can spread thrush.

Instead you need to stop feeding. Actually, it is not possible to bite and actively feed at the same time so you will not be interrupting her if you:

- Remove her from your breast immediately (using your little finger to break the suction, otherwise you could hurt your nipple even more).
- Say 'no' or 'no biting' very firmly.
- Put her on the floor.
- Keep doing this until she gets the message.

Some babies bite anything when they are teething. If you think that this is the problem:

- Give her a chilled teething ring and let her have a good chew on that before a feed.

If you think she is frustrated or angry about something, try to find the reason. This also applies to any baby who has been feeding happily for some time and then suddenly starts fighting or refusing the breast. Possible explanations include:

- A strong flavour in your milk, because of something unusual that you have eaten, for example, garlic or other spices. A lot of alcohol may also change the taste of breast milk. (See box on page 61: 'Was it something I ate?')
- Hormones – if your periods start again or you get pregnant, hormones can get through to the breast milk and change its taste.
- Your baby might have a cold, and is finding it hard to breathe through her nose.
- Teething – milk teeth can push through at any time after birth (even before) and make your baby's gums swollen and painful during feeding.

- Thrush could be making your baby's mouth sore, making it uncomfortable for her to feed.
- Earache – ear pain can spread to the jaw. Ear infections may also cause vomiting, a high temperature and general irritability.
- Loss of appetite – sometimes babies just go off their food for a while.

Keep offering your baby the breast while you think about possible causes: many of these are temporary problems. Although it is frustrating and you may feel as though you and your milk are being rejected, you will find a way through this.

Try the following:
- Exclude any unusual foods from your diet, to see whether this is affecting your milk.
- Check your feeding position and your baby's nose. If it is blocked ask your doctor for nose drops.
- Rub teething powders on your baby's gums before you start to feed, or let her chew on a teething gel ring that has been in the fridge.
- Check for signs of thrush (see page 35) and see your doctor for treatment.
- See your doctor if you think your baby has an ear infection or another illness. Paracetamol syrup can help reduce your baby's pain; antibiotics are not always necessary.
- Stay as calm as you can when you try to feed. If you have other children, get someone to help with them while you concentrate on your baby.

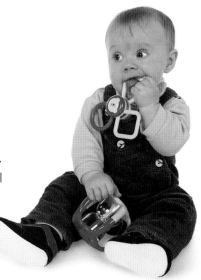

Above: Some babies will bite anything when they are teething.

special situations

- Flat or inverted nipples

- Breast problems

- Illness in the mother

- Twins and triplets

5

- Caesarean section

- Premature babies

- Tongue-tied babies

- Jaundice in newborn babies

Flat or inverted nipples

Although 97 per cent of women can breastfeed, some special situations can make it difficult to get started. Fortunately, with the right help and advice, most of these problems can be overcome.

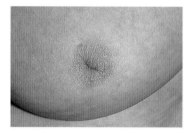

Above: *Women with inverted nipples can breastfeed successfully.*

About 2 per cent of women have inverted nipples that go inward when the areola is pressed. A further 5–8 per cent have flat nipples that do not stand out or become erect when they are cold or stimulated.

During pregnancy you can do various exercises or wear breast shells to encourage your nipples to stand out, but research shows that this makes little difference. Nevertheless, many women with inverted nipples can breastfeed effectively. What counts is not the shape of the nipple but how stretchy the skin around it is and how easily your baby can draw it out to make a teat.

- Learn how to hand express (see page 84) – expressed colostrum can be given in a syringe.
- When your milk comes in, use a hand pump before a feed to draw out the nipple.
- In extreme situations only, and using skilled help, use nipple shields to draw your nipples out at the beginning of a feed.
- Get help positioning your baby so that he gets a good latch.
- If necessary, express milk and cup-feed for a few weeks – breastfeeding may become easier when your baby is older.

Breast problems

Some women worry about the effects of breast size or surgery on their success at breastfeeding. In fact, both of these rarely cause any problems.

Big breasts

If you have large breasts, you may need to support the weight of the breast at every feed. Otherwise, you cannot see what you are doing and the breast may rest on your baby's chin or nose.

- Ask a breastfeeding counsellor to show you how to support the breast so that it does not interfere with feeding or put pressure on any area – which could cause a blocked duct (see page 32).

Breast surgery

Whether you can breastfeed after surgery depends on whether any milk ducts or major nerves were cut or damaged. If milk ducts were cut, this can affect the amount of milk a baby gets from that breast, although the duct system may have healed itself so you may still be able to make milk. If nerves were cut, the baby's sucking on the nipple and areola may not stimulate the brain to produce the hormones that make and release the milk. If the surgery involved only one breast, you should be able to breastfeed normally exclusively from the other breast.

- Contact your surgeon, explain your wish to breastfeed, and find out how the surgery may have affected the nerves and milk ducts.
- If you have any doubts, be especially vigilant in the early days to make sure your baby is getting enough milk (see page 38).
- If you are planning breast surgery it may be possible for the surgeon to avoid damage to major nerves and milk ducts.

Silicone breast implants

Women who have silicone breast implants can still breastfeed, but studies looking at possible risks for babies have had mixed results. For example, a study in 1998 found that levels of silicone in breast milk were much the same whether a woman had implants or not. However, other, very small studies have shown possible side-effects. Research is underway to establish whether the polyurethane coating used on some implants can break down and release potentially harmful chemicals. Meanwhile, the benefits of breastfeeding may still outweigh the risks and women who have had implants should get advice from their doctors.

Illness in the mother

Being ill when you have a young baby is no joke. If you are seriously ill you may not feel like breastfeeding or believe it to be safe for your baby. But, it's worth thinking through this situation as you may have more options than you thought.

Contraceptive pills

If you want to use a contraceptive pill, the progestogen-only pill (the mini pill) is best. The combined pill is not recommended for breastfeeding women, because it reduces milk volume. Although the mini pill hormones do pass into breast milk there are no known dangers from this. Breastfeeding does lower your chances of getting pregnant but it is not 100 per cent reliable.

In fact, if you are ill but want to continue breastfeeding, this is usually only a problem if you are taking medication that is unsuitable for your baby (see below). If you want to stop breastfeeding until you recover or finish your course of drugs, you can express milk to keep up your supply. If you have a cough, cold or flu, your baby will already have been exposed to the infection by the time you show symptoms.

Continuing to breastfeed is actually the best thing you can do, because your baby will get huge amounts of antibodies in the milk. If you have diarrhoea and vomiting as a result of food poisoning, it is usually safe to continue feeding unless you become so ill that you need antibiotics (see below). Remember that if you stop feeding suddenly, your breasts will get painfully engorged and you could end up with mastitis to add to your existing illness.

- If you have a fever or you have been sick, drink more to avoid dehydration.
- Be very careful with hygiene.
- Consult your doctor.
- Get someone to help you, so that you can rest.
- If you feel too ill to continue feeding all the time, try to keep one or two feeds so that your breasts do not get so engorged.
- Do not panic if you have to stop breastfeeding – it should be possible to start again (see Questions and answers, page 92).

Breastfeeding while taking medicines

Almost any drug you take will get into your breast milk in small amounts, but very few prescription drugs or over-the-counter medicines pose any risk to a breastfed baby.

Always:

- Read the label carefully or ask the pharmacist.
- Tell your doctor that you are breastfeeding before he or she starts to prescribe!

If the drug normally prescribed is not compatible with breastfeeding, there is usually an alternative. Your doctor can consult a drug-reference book, which you could ask to see. However, the safety information is often very cautious, for example: 'The drug passes into breast milk. Discuss with your doctor' or 'At normal doses adverse effects on the baby are unlikely'.

If you are not confident that a drug which you need is safe, and there is no alternative, you could either express and discard your milk while you are taking the drug or delay treatment while you double pump to build up a store of frozen milk for your baby when you do start taking it.

Another option is to work out a schedule of drug-taking and feeding that minimizes the amount of drug that could pass into your breastmilk – a once-a-day pill before your baby's longest sleep, for example. You would need to discuss this with your doctor to find out how the drug works and how quickly it is cleared from your system.

Street drugs

Street drugs, such as cocaine and marijuana, should never be taken by breastfeeding mothers because they pose serious risks for babies. Cocaine in breast milk causes vomiting and diarrhoea. It also makes babies irritable and raises their blood pressure and heart rate. Marijuana in breast milk can make a baby sleepy and unable to feed properly, which can lead to weight loss. It may also delay a baby's development.

Below: If you have a cough, cold or flu, your baby should remain healthy if you continue to breastfeed – in fact, she will receive huge amounts of antibodies from your milk.

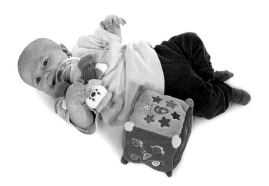

Twins and triplets

Women expecting twins or triplets need to think carefully about the way they will feed their babies. Breastfeeding is demanding but does have advantages.

'I really was determined but I wasn't prepared for how different the girls would be. Sophie latched on straightaway and always fed really well but Emily was very fussy and because of that I couldn't feed them at the same time. So it took forever to get them both fed and I did sometimes feel quite resentful towards Emily, which was terrible. But luckily my mum was able to stay for the whole of the first month so I could take Emily into a quiet room and really concentrate. It took several weeks before she could feed well and then I managed to get them going together, which was brilliant. You do need help though.'

Lorna West, mother of twin girls Sophie and Emily (3 years), had great plans to breastfeed.

Breastfeeding more than one baby may seem a daunting task and it will be very time-consuming – unless you can manage to breastfeed two babies at the same time. Avoiding formula should keep your babies healthier, which will be time-saving in the long run. In practice, many mothers of multiples use a mixture of bottles and breast, often putting formula milk in the bottle – but if you are determined to give your babies nothing but breast milk it can be done. It may help if you:

- Get to know your local breastfeeding counsellor and enlist her help both before and after the birth – ask for advice on positions for double feeding and expressing.
- Tell everyone (and yourself) that you are going to concentrate on the babies and nothing else for the first month.
- Get help with housework, shopping and cooking so you can achieve this.
- Breastfeed early and express milk if you need to be separated from one or more babies in the early days.
- Avoid dummies early on so that you build up a good supply of milk.
- Hire or buy a double pump so that you can express milk for other people to give in bottles after the babies are a month old. In this way you can get a rest at times!

Caesarean section

Women who give birth by caesarean section should certainly encounter no problems and be able to breastfeed their babies, bearing in mind a few things.

There are two special considerations when starting to breastfeed after a caesarean:
- Delay before the first feed.
- Lifting your baby up and finding the most comfortable position.

If you have had a general anaesthetic, there may be a delay while you recover.
- Make sure that the midwife knows you intend to breastfeed, and that your partner knows your baby should not be given formula.
- Put your baby to the breast as soon as you feel able – the earlier he starts to feed, the better.
- Ask someone to put the baby to your breast.

You will probably find it impossible to lift your baby without help. This is because your stomach muscles have been separated during the operation. Sitting up to feed and laying the baby on your lap can also be uncomfortable.
- Ask for help and use the call bell!
- Ask a breastfeeding counsellor to advise you on feeding while you are lying down or using the football hold – with your baby beneath your arm with arms and legs tucked in – if it is uncomfortable to have the baby on your lap.
- Whichever position you choose, use plenty of pillows and cushions for support.
- Ask a midwife or obstetric physiotherapist to show you how to sit up and move from side to side.
- Use the pain relief offered.

Milk coming in

You may hear people say that it takes longer for milk to come in after a caesarean section. If this happens, it is probably because the mother is feeling uncomfortable and so feeding is less frequent.

Epidurals and spinal blocks

If you have had an epidural or spinal block, whether during either a normal delivery or a caesarean section, you should still be able to feed your baby straightaway, but you may need someone to support the baby as you will probably have to lie on your back for a while.

Premature babies

Breastmilk has important benefits for all babies but is particularly important for babies who are born very early.

Right: *Premature babies may need to be fed your breastmilk through a tube.*

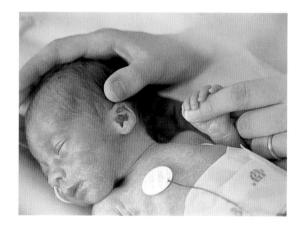

Any baby born 3 or more weeks early is classified as premature, or 'prem', although many are strong, healthy, feed well and need no special treatment. However, a premature baby may need help with breathing or may need to be tube-fed until he is able to suck. This may also be necessary if he is receiving special care. Whenever your baby is born, your body will make the most perfect food for him: premature baby milk is different from full-term baby milk. It is full of proteins and antibodies that are vital if he is frail and important to his continued development. Research has shown that premature babies fed with breast milk have a higher IQ than those fed on formula.

Expressing milk for tube-feeding and spending time touching your baby are among the best things you can do for him. You can also:

Getting breastfeeding established for premature babies

- Have someone with you to help you position and hold the baby, such as a midwife or breastfeeding counsellor.
- Follow the guidelines for latching on (see page 14).
- Support your baby's head and your breast if he is small.
- Use a pump or hand massage to stimulate your let-down reflex before your baby latches on.
- Get support and encouragement from your partner, friends and family. You will need this to persevere.
- Try expressing some milk directly into your baby's mouth.
- Continue expressing after and even between feeds if your baby is feeding for short periods. This milk can be given in a cup or through a tube until he is able to feed for longer. It is important to keep up your supply.
- Get the support of a breastfeeding counsellor once you get home. Most mothers feel a bit unsure at first, especially if their baby has been in hospital for a long time. Call a breastfeeding helpline for advice or reassurance.

- Hold your baby – skin-to-skin contact will help your let-down, even if you go on to pump afterwards. Research shows that women who do this tend to breastfeed for longer.
- Express more milk than he needs – the extra can be frozen. Although fresh milk is best, if your

'Although he was fine, he was very small and couldn't suck, so he went into special care for 2 weeks. The midwife actually asked me to express some colostrum as soon as he was born and I was happy to do that because I wanted to breastfeed. I have to say it was quite hard work getting the colostrum out but it did get easier and soon I was double pumping. It was fantastic taking the bottles into the unit and watching the milk go along the tube and into his nose. I felt so proud I could do that for him. When he was a bit stronger I started to get him up and let him nuzzle at the breast a few times each day. I was warned not to expect him to feed straightaway and it did take quite a few attempts but it was lovely to hold him and I felt confident he was getting the milk he needed through the tube. Eventually he did start to suck and I breastfed him for 9 months.'

Julia Braithwaite gave birth to her son Timothy 6 weeks early.

baby is going to be in special care for a while you may want to spend some time away from the hospital. Expressing will also help to build up your supply.

Expressing breast milk takes time and practice and you are unlikely to get more than a few drops the first few times. Once your milk has come in, double pumping with an electric pump is usually most efficient (see page 85), but find a method with which you feel comfortable. You will need to express about eight times over a 24-hour period. If your baby does not gain weight, the doctors may want to supplement your milk with other nutrients. Other ways to increase his weight gain are to:

- Increase the amount of breastmilk you give him at each feed.
- Give the fat-rich hindmilk, discarding the foremilk.

Establishing breastfeeding

The more premature your baby, the longer it will take to establish breastfeeding. However, there is no need for premature babies to go from tube-feeding to bottle-feeding with expressed breast milk before trying the breast. In fact, using bottles in this transitional period reduces the establishment of breastfeeding and studies have shown that babies find it easier to breastfeed than to bottle-feed. By going straight to the breast you will avoid nipple confusion (see page 80–81). Alternatively your baby could go from tube- to cup-feeding if he has initial problems latching on or only breastfeeds for very short periods. Cup-feeding teaches a baby how to use his tongue and gets him used to controlling milk in his mouth. Once your baby is breastfeeding you can feed on demand – there is no need to keep to the schedule used in the special-care unit.

Tongue-tied babies

For a few babies there are anatomical reasons why feeding is difficult – such as tongue tie, short tongue or cleft lip and palate.

Babies who are tongue-tied have a short frenulum – the tissue attaching the tongue to the floor of the mouth. This may cause problems with breastfeeding if the baby's tongue cannot grasp and milk the breast. The same is true of babies with a short tongue. This can lead to:
- Sore nipples.
- Frequent feeding.
- Problems getting the baby onto the breast.
- Fussiness – constant coming off and on the breast.
- Slow weight gain.
- Poor milk supply.
- Mastitis.

Any problem may resolve itself as the baby grows and his tongue stretches. If not, or if you are concerned:
- A breastfeeding counsellor may be able to suggest improvements to your feeding position.
- Your doctor can clip the frenulum – this can be done in the surgery and does not involve an anaesthetic.

Babies with cleft lip and palate

Although cleft lip and palate are distressing for parents, corrective surgery is very successful. A cleft lip can be repaired when the baby is only 48 hours old, although a cleft palate may have to wait for 6–12 months. Both can cause feeding problems: a severe cleft palate may make it impossible for the baby to feed but he can have breast milk in a cup or special bottle, or through a tube.

- Ask a breastfeeding counsellor to help you find a position in which your baby can feed successfully.

- Express milk for cup- or tube-feeding.

- Start breastfeeding early after surgery: research shows there is no need to wait (to protect the wound).

Jaundice in newborn babies

One in two newborn babies develops jaundice: as the immature liver struggles to process the products of normal red cell breakdown there is a build-up of bilirubin in the blood, which produces yellowing of the skin and the whites of the eyes a couple of days after birth. Babies do not need any treatment for this unless the bilirubin levels rise too high, but jaundice can make a baby sleepy and reluctant to feed.

Right: *Babies with jaundice need light therapy to help bring down their bilirubin levels.*

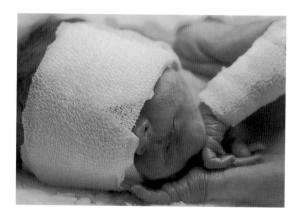

- Persevere, and try to give your baby a feed every couple of hours (see page 42). As the liver matures the jaundice should resolve and, in the meantime, she needs the fluids that she gets from your milk. Frequent breastfeeding helps, particularly in the first 48 hours, because colostrum has a natural laxative effect. It shifts the meconium in the gut, which contains bilirubin that might otherwise be reabsorbed into the baby's blood.
- Do not limit your baby's feeding.

Babies with hypoglycaemia

Hypoglycaemia, or low blood sugar, occurs when the body is using glucose faster than it produces it. This can make a baby lethargic, limp, sweaty, jittery and difficult to feed. Some babies who are ill, premature, small for dates or born to diabetic mothers may suffer from low blood sugar and need special treatment. They can still breastfeed, but may need other feeds as well. Other babies may have hypoglycaemia because they do not feed very well in the early days. However, it is more likely to be caused by an underlying illness and supplementary feeds are not always the answer. A baby with low blood sugar should be examined and observed while you:

• Increase the number of feeds you give.

• Express and give extra breast milk in a cup or via a tube.

• Put your baby in the light – this will help to bring down the bilirubin levels.

If a baby is born jaundiced or jaundice occurs on the first day, however, this indicates that she has a blood condition requiring treatment. This is because, if the levels of bilirubin get too high, she could suffer brain damage. Therefore, when jaundice does not clear up after a day or too, babies are given heel-prick blood tests to monitor their bilirubin levels. If levels get too high, the baby will be given phototherapy – treatment with ultraviolet light – which breaks down the bilirubin pigment in the skin. Most modern maternity units use a biliblanket – a blanket that delivers light while it is wrapped around the baby.

Breastfeeding can still continue unless the baby has a very rare condition that means she is unable to digest the lactose in milk. There is rarely any need for your baby to be given formula milk as a supplement and, if you feel under pressure to accept this, you should:

• Contact your breastfeeding counsellor.

• Express milk to build up your supply: if your baby has not fed frequently in the first few days then your supply may not be enough for her yet (see page 38).

hello bottle:
introducing bottles and formula

- Introducing the first bottle
- Dropping feeds
- Expressing milk

6

- Giving formula milk

- Weaning

Introducing the first bottle

Breast and bottle-feeding involve different sucking techniques so you will need to plan the introduction of bottles carefully.

Differences between breastfeeding and bottle-feeding

Breastfeeding	Bottle-feeding
Mouth open wide	Mouth only slightly open
Whole jaw involved in sucking	Jaw still
Lips flanged and fairly still	Lips do most of the work
Tongue 'strips' the breast	Tongue relatively still
Delay before let-down	No waiting – milk flows

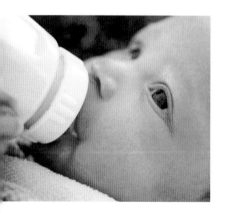

Above: *Breastfed babies may need time to get used to bottle-feeding.*

Some breastfed babies love bottles. They simply love drinking, and do not mind where the milk comes from or how it arrives. Others are very fussy and are only happy when they have the same thing served up in the same way every time. Most babies fall somewhere between these two extremes, but many women who have been breastfeeding report at least some difficulty getting their babies to take to feeding from a bottle.

The most obvious explanation for this is that breastfed babies enjoy breastfeeding: they like the skin-to-skin contact and listening to their mother's heartbeat, as well as the really close cuddle that comes with it. They also quickly get used to the smell and taste of their mother's breast milk, the rate at which it flows and the control they have over that flow.

With the best technology in the world, a silicone teat is not going to feel exactly the same as a human nipple. What is more, if a baby has been breastfed from birth, it is a major part of his life and giving food in another form could represent a threat to him. Babies can learn to love bottle-feeding too, of course, but they will need time to get used to the change.

Possible solutions are to:

- Start fairly early once breastfeeding is well established.
- Put breast milk in bottles so that the milk at least tastes the same.
- Do it slowly, one feed at a time.
- Consider delaying your return to work until your baby is fully weaned and he is less reliant on milk for nutrition.
- Work short part-time hours – most babies can manage 3 hours without a drink.

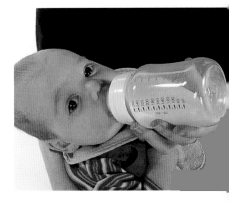

Above: *If possible delay giving a bottle until after three weeks, to avoid confusing your baby.*

When?

There is no absolute right or wrong time to give a breastfed baby his first bottle, but expert advice is that you should not be too hasty: if you give it in the first 3 weeks – before you really have breastfeeding established – you could reduce your milk supply and confuse your baby. This is because breast-feeding and bottle-feeding involve two quite different techniques (see table, above left).

Dropping feeds

If you want to move from exclusive breastfeeding to mixed feeding – using some bottles as well – you will need to plan the change carefully.

Sterilizing equipment

It is vitally important to sterilize all the equipment used in making up a bottle – teats, lids, bottles, spoons – the lot. Gastroenteritis – a tummy bug – is much more common in bottle-fed babies and hygiene is an important factor in this. You can sterilize using tablets, or in a micro-wave or steam sterilizer.

If you know that you are going to return to work or you just want the occasional day off, you could try introducing one bottle every few days after your baby is a month old. Some experts think you should introduce the first bottle before 6 weeks.

Unfortunately, even if your baby does take a bottle early on, it is no absolute guarantee that he will do so when he is older. For this reason, some women do not bother trying until a couple of weeks before they return to work. The worst case scenario is that your baby refuses bottles and you have to leave him without a major source of liquid when you return to work.

In practice, most babies will drink if they are thirsty, even if it is in small amounts. You may find that you need to feed more in the evenings and at night to compensate. You could also consider delaying your return to work until your baby is fully weaned and less reliant on milk for nutrition – or working short hours for a few months. There is a chance that your baby might prefer the bottle and reject the breast, but the longer your baby has been breastfed the less likely this is.

How?

If you have definitely decided to give formula, then it might be better if someone else gave the first few bottles – if you are holding your baby he is likely to smell the breast milk and start rooting after it. If you are giving breast milk in the bottle, it may not matter who gives it. If it does not work first time:

- Keep trying once a day for just a few minutes.
- Do not expect him to take the whole feed – even 28g (1oz) is a positive sign.
- Give the bottle before he is really hungry.
- Do not push the teat into the baby's mouth – let it touch his lips so that he reaches for it.
- Warm and soften the teat with boiled water.
- Try giving the bottle to your baby while he is in a bouncy chair.
- Look at alternative teats: there are several different shapes made from silicone or rubber with different numbers of holes to alter the flow.
- Try a lidded cup or beaker instead – even 3-month-old babies may be able to cope with this.

Dropping feeds

If you drop too many feeds at once your breasts will become painfully full. Allow several days or even a week between each feed that you drop. It may help if you do not do this at the same time as introducing bottles: it could be agony for you and your baby if your breasts are dripping with milk and you are trying to insist that he has formula from a bottle!

'With both of them I tried giving one bottle when they were only 4 or 5 weeks old and because they seemed happy with it I assumed they'd be fine when I wanted to start bottles seriously at about 4 months. It worked with Toby but Andrew refused to have anything to do with teats – he only wanted nipples! He used to scream and fuss and push the teat out. In the end I just left him with a childminder for a few hours during which time he coped without a drink. Then when he was about 6 months old I had got him to take water or expressed milk from a cup. Ironically when he was 8 months old I tried again and he took to bottles really easily!'

Karen Smart, mother of Toby (5 years) and Andrew (2 years), found it very difficult to get one of her babies interested in bottles.

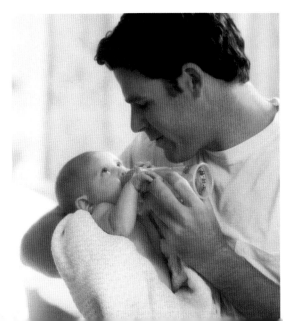

Left: *It may help if someone else gives the first bottle.*

Expressing milk

If you want to give breast milk in bottles, you will need to learn how to express your milk. You can do this by hand or using a pump. Either way, expressing is a skill and you will need to practice. It won't just happen the first time! In fact, you may spend half an hour getting a few drops. Do not give up!

Tips for expressing milk

- Get yourself comfortable, warm and relaxed before you start.
- Warm your breasts with a warm flannel.
- Massage your breasts and stimulate the nipples.
- Think about your baby.

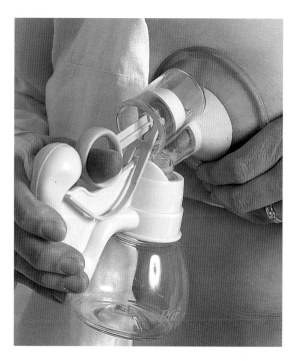

Right: A good pump will draw out the nipple and stimulate the let-down reflex with strong suction.

- Do it in the morning, just after a feed, when you are feeling full or when you have a spontaneous let-down.
- Ask a breastfeeding counsellor for help with your technique if you want to express by hand.
- Try different pumps (see below) – different brands work for different women and, even if you are pleased with the one you have, it is worth seeing if there is something more suitable for you.

Storing breast milk

If it is expressed into sterilized containers and you are careful with hygiene, breast milk can be stored for long periods.

- **At room temperature (20–25°C):** 4 hours.
- **In a cooler with icepacks:** 24 hours.
- **In a fridge (0–4°C):** 2 days or more.
- **In a freezer:** 3 months and then 24 hours in a fridge.

It is important to label containers with the date you express the milk. You can top-up bottles with further expressed milk but always go by the expiry time of the first batch. Small amounts of frozen milk can be useful because they are easier to thaw and heat through, and there is less waste. Always let fresh milk cool for 30 minutes before adding to frozen milk. Never refreeze thawed milk.

Choosing a pump

If you are returning to work and want to express serious amounts of milk every day, it might be worth investing in an electric pump with a double collection set. This means that you can just switch on and milk is expressed from both breasts in about 15 minutes. If you use a hand pump or hand express milk, it could take twice as long and involve a lot more physical effort. You might also be able to hire an electric pump, which is useful if you only need it for odd days or if you want to try it out before you buy it.

Expressing essentials

- A good pump
- Sterilized containers and labels
- A cool bag and ice packs, or a special feeding bag with a cooler section
- Access to a fridge and a freezer compartment
- Sterilizing equipment
- Hot water, washing-up liquid, a towel and soap
- Access to a quiet, private room (ideally with a lock, a sink and a power point)
- A spare t-shirt or top in case of leaks
- Spare batteries
- A kit bag

There are several varieties of pump and you should choose the one that suits you best.

- Hand pumps take time and practice, need physical effort and are tiring. On the other hand, they are cheap and there is no equipment to carry.
- Hand-held pumps, battery- or hand- operated, may need two hands and can be slow, but they are quiet, light, portable and fairly cheap. There is a new-style manual pump that stimulates the breast well and is at least as quick as a single electric pump.
- Automatic pumps, electric or battery-operated, mimic the suction and release patterns of feeding babies. They do not require any skill to operate and are quick to use. However, they are heavier, often less portable, can be noisy and are relatively expensive.

Is it worth it?

If you are returning to work or your baby is taking bottles, you might wonder whether it is worth continuing to breastfeed at all. Remember the advantages:

- Breast milk is the best food for your baby.
- It is something psychologically and emotionally rewarding that only you can do for your baby.
- It will keep you close.

'Most of the time I work from home and I'm lucky to have an au pair. She would call me when Chloe needed feeding and so I was effectively able to go back to work full time when she was only 4 months old. But sometimes I need to go into London for all day meetings, seminars or conferences. Because it was all planned in advance I would hire an electric pump the day before, express extra milk and leave it for Chloe. Then I'd take the pump with me and express during coffee breaks. I only needed to store the milk once, when I was out for two consecutive days but the pump came with a cool bag and it was much more straightforward than I thought it would be.'

Julia Prescott, mother of Chloe (2 years), used a pump to express milk on days when she needed to work in London.

Expressing milk at work

If you want your child to be fully breastfed, even though you are away for most of some days, you will need to express milk every few hours during the day in order to keep up your supply and stop your breasts getting painfully full. Women in the UK have no right to time off for expressing milk or, indeed, to a place to do it in, so you may have to use some persuasion. It may help to point out to your employer that breast milk provides your baby with protection against infection and so you will be less likely to take time off to cope with illness. Since your baby's health is at risk if you stop breastfeeding, it is in your employer's interest to take steps to enable you to continue.

Before you start in earnest, have a trial run.

• Build up a store of expressed milk in the freezer to cope with days when you cannot express.
• Wear suitable clothes – a dress is not a good idea!
• Be organized: sterilize your pump and bottles and pack your bag before you go to bed.

If possible, delay returning to work until your baby is at least 16 weeks old or work part time.

'When Philippa was 12 weeks old I needed to go to university one day a week for 6 weeks so I expressed at least one bottle of milk every other day and froze it so she had a day's supply to take to the nursery. She was very accommodating about taking a bottle – it was me who had the problems! I was so uncomfortable by midday I had to go to the health centre to express off a load of milk. After Dominic was born I wanted to go back to playing the flute one night a week with my local orchestra so I was keen to get him taking a bottle. But he wasn't having it. In the end I left it for a while and when I tried again I found it made a real difference using a soft latex teat rather than a hard silicone one. By the time he was 4 or 5 months old I was breastfeeding night and morning and giving bottles of formula during the day.'

Fiona Humphreys, mother of Philippa (3 years) and Dominic (1 year)

Giving formula milk

Giving bottles and giving formula may be separate decisions for you. If breastfeeding and expressions go well your baby may never need formula milk.

Reactions to formula

Your baby is fairly unlikely to have a reaction to formula milk but, if you think he has, note the date, symptoms and the brand you used. Switch to another brand, if you wish. If necessary, your doctor can prescribe a hypoallergenic formula. After 6 months, a baby can have cow's milk in food. After a year, babies can have full-fat cow's milk as their main drink.

There are many different brands of formula milk, each formulated after decades of research to make it as close to breast milk as possible. Based on cow's milk, they contain carbohydrates, fats, protein, minerals and vitamins. No formula milk is exactly the same as breast milk, which is full of live cells and tailored to the individual baby. Your baby can be well fed on formula, but you do need to be quite careful.

- Choose a brand appropriate for your baby's age. Do not give 'follow-on milks' to a baby under 6 months just because he is a big boy. Follow-on milks contain more protein, iron and vitamin D.
- Follow instructions carefully. Do not be tempted to add extra powder or to dilute milk. During hot weather, if your baby is having lots of formula and seems very thirsty he could have a drink of cooled, boiled water between feeds. Exclusively breastfed babies do not need water or any other drinks because breast milk adapts to have a higher water content if necessary.
- Be scrupulous about hygiene. Discard any left-over milk.
- Keep a note of the date you open a tin of formula. If you only give the occasional bottle, it might be better to buy a small tin.

Weaning

Weaning means the introduction of 'solid' food into your baby's diet. In fact, the first foods are usually processed to a liquid that is more filling than milk.

Breastfed babies do not need solids before they are 6 months old. Until then, breast milk gives them all they need nutritionally. Research is clear that babies who have nothing but breast milk for 6 months have fewer health problems than babies who start solids earlier. It is not so clear whether this is the same for babies who have a mix of breast and formula milk. What is certain is that no babies should be given solids before they are 4 months old. Why is this?

- It increases their risk of allergies – at 6 months babies produce enough antibodies to fight allergens.
- It can cause digestive problems – the digestive system needs 6 months to mature.
- It increases the risk of ear infections – breast milk contains antibodies that fight infections.
- It is hard and messy – younger babies tend to push food out rather than swallow it and they cannot sit up alone.

When your baby is eating good amounts of solid food you can offer cooled, boiled water as a drink, but only if you are confident that he is getting about a pint of milk a day. Discuss this with your health visitor. Babies do not need fruit juice or squash, which are bad for their teeth.

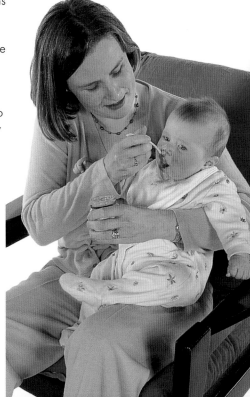

Below: Babies should not be given solids until they are aged at least 4 months.

Troubleshooting chart

Problem	Possible causes	Helpful chapters
Blocked duct	• Ducts not emptying properly, pressure on breasts	2
Biting	• Unable to breathe – positioning problem	1, 4
	• Strong flavours or hormones in milk	4
Breast abscess	• Ineffective treatment for mastitis	2
	• Nipple shields	
Breast refusal	• Baby unable to breathe freely.	1
	• Unhappy memory of being forced to feed.	
	• Slow or forceful let-down	
Colic	• Check positioning	1, 4
	• Temporary lactose overload	4
Cracked and bleeding nipples	• Check positioning (see Sore nipples, right)	1, 2
Engorgement	• Increased blood supply as milk comes in	1
	• Feeding infrequently or missing feeds	
Frequent feeding	• Check positioning.	1
	• Normal pattern or growth spurt.	
	• Illness	
Leaking	• Normal over-supply in first 6 weeks.	1
	• Check positioning	
Mastitis	• Blocked duct (see left).	1, 2
	• Check positioning	

Problem	Possible causes	Helpful chapters
Milk supply	• Check positioning. • Anxiety. • Giving bottles • Growth spurt	1 3
Reluctant feeder	• Sleepy baby. • Pethidine hangover • Jaundice. • Hypoglycaemia • Uncomfortable baby	3 3, 5 4
Slow growth	• Nipple-feeding. • Feeding infrequently. • Medical condition	3
Sore breasts	• Check positioning • Thrush	1 2
Sore nipples	• Check positioning • Thrush. • Sensitivity to soaps/creams	1, 2 2
Vomiting	• Gulping air – check positioning • Illness. • Reflux. • Cow's milk intolerance. • Pyloric stenosis. Hernia	1, 4 4

Right: If your baby seems unhappy or uncomfortable, it could be for one of several reasons. The troubleshooting chart above should help.

Problem-solving
questions and answers

Q **If I stop breastfeeding my baby can I change my mind and start again later?**

A Yes – although, depending on when you stop and restart, it can take a month or more to rebuild your milk supply. As long as your baby cooperates, you can restart after almost any interval. The more often you put your baby to the breast, the more milk you will produce. You might also speed things up by expressing milk between feeds. It may take your baby some time to get used to breastfeeding again because bottle-feeding involves a different sucking technique (see table, page 80). A breastfeeding counsellor will be able to help you.

Q **Should I stop breastfeeding my baby if she has diarrhoea?**

A No – but it is important that you should see your doctor, particularly if your baby is vomiting as well. Note how many dirty nappies your baby produces and keep a couple to show your doctor. The danger with ordinary diarrhoea is dehydration (see page 45), so it's important to go on feeding. Breast milk is easily digested – unlike formula milk – and won't prolong your baby's recovery time. Your doctor may recommend a rehydration powder that can be given by spoon or cup. If your baby's nappies are green and frothy, see a breast-feeding counsellor for advice – there could be a problem with your feeding position (see page 14).

Below: Artificial teats involve a different sucking technique, which your baby can learn.

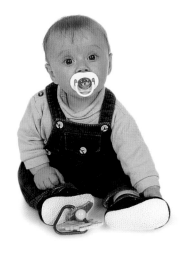

Q I expressed some milk and put it in the fridge but after 12 hours it seemed to have gone off – why?

A If left to stand, breast milk separates into different layers and can look blue or yellow – but it won't have gone off. It will keep for at least 2 days at 0–4°C. If you are not sure, smell and taste it. Defrosted frozen milk can smell soapy, so give it a shake before you warm it up.

Q I can't find a pump that suits me although I have tried several. Am I just unable to express milk?

A This is unlikely to be the case. First check that you have followed all the expressing tips – when and where you pump as well as how you are feeling may be as important as the pump itself. Most women can express with an electric pump. Contact a breastfeeding counsellor who hires out electric pumps, and ask for her help.

Q How much milk do I need to express for a feed?

A There are no absolute guidelines in terms of ounces of milk: those on a formula tin relate to formula, not to breast milk. In general, express from both breasts twice. Stop when the amount slows, have a break and start again. If you are expressing instead of feeding your baby, this should give you enough milk for a full feed. If you are expressing after a feed, you will get less milk and may need to express again later and combine the two to get enough for one feed.

Index

a

abscesses, 30, 33, 34
afterpains, 22, 23
alcohol, 49, 61, 62
allergies, 60–1, 89
alveoli, 11
anaesthesia, 71
anhydrous lanolin,, 30, 31
antibiotics, 31, 33, 34, 63, 68
antibodies, 10, 13, 38, 61, 68, 72, 89
anxiety, breast refusal, 20–1
appetite, loss of, 63
areola, latching on, 14, 16–17

b

bacteria, 33, 56
bilirubin, 40–1, 76–7
birthweight, 44, 46
biting nipples, 62–3
bleeding, 30–1, 34
blocked ducts, 32
blood-sugar levels, 41, 77
boredom, 53
bottle-feeding:
  formula milk, 88
  growth rates, 47
  hypoallergenic formula, 61, 88
  introducing, 80–3
  premature babies, 74
  supplementary feeds, 49
brain, control of milk supply, 12
bras, 25, 32
breast milk: benefits of, 10
  cup-feeding, 19, 74
  expressing, 49, 84–7
  how much milk?, 38–9
  how often?, 39
  improving supply, 48–9
  let-down reflex, 12, 18, 19, 23, 49
  premature babies, 72

storing, 85, 93
supply and demand, 12
types of, 13
breast pads, 23, 29
breast refusal, 19–21
breast shells, 22, 23, 66
breasts: abscesses, 30, 33, 34
  big breasts, 67
  blocked ducts, 32
  dropping feeds, 83
  engorgement, 22–3, 68
  implants, 67
  leaking, 18, 23, 48–9
  mastitis, 30, 33, 34, 68
  small breasts, 13, 48
  structure, 11
  surgery, 13, 67
  see also nipples
breathing problems, 20
burping, 54, 57

c

caesarean section, 71
caffeine, 49, 61
cleft lip and palate, 75
colds, 62, 68
colic, 55–6, 58, 61
colostrum, 13, 18, 38, 42, 74, 76
coming off and on the breast, 18
contraceptive pills, 68
counsellors, breastfeeding, 18, 28, 58
cow's milk, 88
  intolerance, 45, 60–1
cracked nipples, 30–1
cranial osteopathy, 21, 58
crying, 52–3, 55, 59
cup-feeding, 19, 74

d

dehydration, 45, 68, 92
diarrhoea, 68, 92
dropping feeds, 83

drugs, 68, 69
ducts, 11
  blocked ducts, 32
  breast surgery, 67
dummies, 43, 59, 62, 70

e

ear infections, 63, 89
engorged breasts, 22–3, 68
epidural anaesthesia, 41, 71
equipment, sterilizing, 82
expressing milk, 49, 70, 73–4, 84–7, 93

f

feeding bras, 25, 32
feeding position, 14–17
fevers, 68
fighting the breast, 62–3
flat nipples, 13, 66
fontanelle, dehydration, 45
forceps delivery, 18
foremilk, 13, 44, 56, 57
formula milk, 88
frequent feeders, 24, 43
fusidic acid, 31

g

gape reflex, 16
gastro-oesophageal reflux, 57
goat's milk, 60
growth rates, 44–7
growth spurts, 24, 49

h

headaches, 58
healing, cracked nipples, 31
hernias, 57
hindmilk, 13, 43, 44, 56
hormones: afterpains, 24
  contraceptive pills, 68
  control of milk supply, 12
  fighting the breast, 62
hypoallergenic formula milk, 61, 88
hypoglycaemia, 41, 77

Picture credits

Bubbles/Frans Rombout 13
/Loisjoy Thurstun 21 left, 58, 84
/Lucy Tizard 10
Corbis UK Ltd/Jose Luis Pelaez 83
Getty Images/Ron Alston 80
/Heath Robbins 43
**Octopus Publishing Group
Limited**/Peter Pugh-Cook 1, 2, 7, 8,
12, 14, 16, 17, 21 right, 23, 25,
26, 28, 29, 32, 35, 36, 39, 40,
42, 45, 46, 47, 52, 53, 54, 55,
56, 59, 60, 63, 69, 81, 89, 91, 92
/William Reavell 48
/Ian Wallace 24, 38

Science Photo Library/Samuel
Ashfield 72
/Tracy Dominey 44
/Mauro Fermariello 76
/Dr. P. Marazzi 31, 66
Gary Winfield 15

About the author

Jane Chumbley is a freelance health writer who specialises in pregnancy and early parenting. She contributes regularly to *Practical Parenting* magazine, is a past health editor for *Bella* magazine and has published several books. Jane is also a qualified antenatal teacher with the National Childbirth Trust and is married with three young children.

Acknowledgements

Many thanks to Adelle Shaw-Flach RGN RHV DPSHV IBCLC for her invaluable and expert help in checking the text, and to all the women who have so willingly shared their breastfeeding experiences with me. Thanks also to Helen Marlow and Wendy Hallett who taught me so much.

Executive Editor: Jane McIntosh
Editors: Abi Rowsell and
Joss Waterfall
Executive Art Editor: Joanna Bennett
Designer: Ginny Zeal
Production Controller:
Lucy Woodhead
Photography: Peter Pugh-Cook
Stylist: Aruna Mathur
With special thanks to Boots The Chemists Ltd for supplying breastfeeding products.